THE HEALING POWER OF PLANETARY METALS

D1557105

THE HEALING POWER
of PLANETARY METALS

in Anthroposophic and Homeopathic Medicine

HENNING M. SCHRAMM

Lindisfarne Books | 2013

LINDISFARNE BOOKS
An imprint of SteinerBooks / Anthroposophic Press, Inc.
610 Main St., Great Barrington, MA 01230
www.steinerbooks.org

Cover and design: William Jens Jensen

LIBRARY OF CONGRESS CONTROL NUMBER: 2013950969

ISBN: 978-1-58420-157-1 (paperback)
ISBN: 978-1-58420-158-8 (ebook)

CONTENTS

INTRODUCTION

The Two Aims of this Study

The purpose of this study of remedies is twofold. The first is to offer a living, imaginative picture of the metallic remedies of anthroposophic and homeopathic medicine. Attempting to understand these remedies through methods of conventional scientific medicine would be inappropriate; it is interested only in the "active" ingredients or principles of remedies—the bioactive chemical substances that interfere with molecular pathways of the organism's cells. In contrast to chemical, agent-based medicine, anthroposophic remedies are based on a paradigm that focuses on *processes* and spiritual-evolutionary relationships. Therefore, we need a means of describing them that is different from what would be appropriate for biochemical agents. In this study, we find that means in fairy-tale imaginations. Fairy-tale imaginations allow us to recognize spiritual efficacies in their lawfulness. They make it possible to develop the kind of understanding that matches the nature of these remedies. In other words, our attempt to approach remedies through fairy tales is not simply a way of recasting abstract, scientific information in a form more accessible and interesting to the reader; it is the essentially appropriate approach for the remedies we are considering.

The therapeutic qualities of the seven chief or solar metals have already been thoroughly described by other authors. Their insights will complement our use of fairy tales to develop a character image of each metal that reveals its inherent connection to the human being and human diseases. Fairy tales make it possible to characterize the metals in a truly comprehensive way, capturing their whole dynamic range and therapeutic vitality. This could never be achieved with an approach based purely on abstract concepts. Nevertheless, how can we prove our interpretations without recourse to scientific abstractions? In fact, it does not matter whether the particular interpretations and characterizations offered here can be "proved" in that way or not. They can be verified only by experience and through the insights of Spiritual Science. The important thing is that they are coherent and that one can work with them in therapeutic practice; these are the only valid criteria for judging the usefulness of our approach.

The other part of our purpose is to demonstrate that the kind of imaginations found in fairy tales have broad significance in and of themselves. Simply occupying oneself with them can be a genuine help in life. Both research and experience confirm that practicing imagination can have a healing action whose effects extend to the physiological processes of the body. Working with imaginations is of particular significance in our times, as we will see from the following discussion.

In our study we interpret fairy-tale imaginations on three different levels—that of the planetary spheres, that of metal processes, and that of human soul qualities. In this way they offer us a marvelous holistic picture of the action of the metals in therapy.

The Common Origin of Fairy Tales and Remedy Pictures

This study explores the remarkable correspondences between specific fairy tales and the remedy pictures of anthroposophic and homeopathic medicine. In some cases, the correspondences are obvious from the beginning. In "Iron Hans," for example, the title itself hints at the deeper aspect of its images; and these images display a clear connection to the homeopathic and anthroposophic drug picture of iron, which will be described later in detail.

The thesis of our study is that these correspondences are not accidental but point to a *common origin*. How is this to be understood?

We may suppose that the originators of fairy tales possessed faculties of clairvoyance, but this explanation remains vague. What can account for a relationship so exact that a certain fairy tale will correspond in all of its motifs, down to the minutest details, to the effects of a certain natural substance in the human being? This only begins to make sense if we take seriously Steiner's indication that those who gave birth to the fairy tales had first ingested specific substances in high dilution. The experiences of homeopathic doctors who develop drug pictures offer a clue to how this could take place. In self-experimentation, homeopathic doctors today take in a highly potentized substance such as iron or gold, and then note the physiological and psychic alterations in themselves, which may also play into one's dream life. Similarly, the originators of fairy tales—considered then to be initiates—would take in such substances to reach inner experiences of a very specific kind. By ingesting potentized iron, for example, adepts would enter a kind of waking dream with a series of images that they would be able to retain and pass on—images that a later age would come to know as the story "Iron Hans." I am personally acquainted with homeopathic doctors who, after taking in a substance in high potency, dreamed particular motifs that we connect here with the very fairy tale whose images represent that potentized substance. If this is still possible today for certain highly trained individuals, it seems likely to have been possible in earlier periods of human development, when the constitution of human beings was much more permeable to spiritual influences. This hypothesis may explain why fairy tales can demonstrate such a close relationship to the natural substances that are used as potentized remedies, as we postulate in this book.

As a cautionary note, it should be pointed out that not every person who takes in highly potentized substances will have spiritual experiences or meaningful dreams. It takes not only a certain physical and psychological constitution, but also special training for this to happen. This is why we suspect that part of the training in the ancient initiation centers entailed conscious cultivation of a faculty that enabled pupils to have spiritual experiences corresponding to genuine fairy-tale images when they ingested highly potentized substances.

With this discussion, the nature of the common origin has become clear; the birth of fairy tales and the development of homeopathic drug pictures both arise from the interaction—or the "crosstalk"—of a potentized substance with the individual human organism. In our attempt to understand this interaction, we shall explore the homeopathic drug pictures connected with each metal as well as the anthroposophic insights into its spiritual dimensions. We shall also look at phenomenological aspects of each metal, but it will not be possible to consider the vast fund of scientific data as well, such as the role of iron in human physiological and molecular processes. This is not because such information is less important than that gained by the imaginative approach, but simply because it goes beyond the scope of the present study.

Two Opposing Theories of Knowledge

The interaction of metal and organism cannot be understood unless we recognize that our organism is not only an *instrument* for understanding the inner and outer world in a scientific way, but also the *source* of this understanding. We are accustomed to another view of knowledge, namely that it comes from the outside and enters us through our senses. This view is by no means so old, nor was it accepted as obvious in former times. It was not until the eighteenth century that John Locke, in Dutch exile, postulated this view of knowledge acquisition in his famous "Essay Concerning Human Understanding." He was the first to propose that man comes into the world as a *tabula rasa*—a blank slate. According to Locke, everything we are conscious of comes into us first through our senses. The initially blank slate begins to fill up through our experiences. The assumption is that we bring no knowledge with us into the world and are accordingly unable to draw it out of ourselves. Everything must first be taken in through the senses.

This view appears so obvious to us today that we do not even wonder if other ways of acquiring knowledge exist. Normally it does not occur to us to consider if our organism might hold inner sources of knowledge. In former times in Europe this was believed to be possible, and today there are still cultures, Buddhist in particular, in which this view is the norm. Even today there are Buddhist institutions of higher learning that are monasteries. What is taught there is not a body of knowledge but an attitude toward life that is conducive to meditation, through which spiritual knowledge can be acquired. The students draw this knowledge out of themselves. Through meditation they access sources of knowledge within. In earlier times this was accepted in Europe as well—when monasteries had the character of universities.

The Inner Path of Scientific Knowledge

The connection between our organism and our cognitive faculties was described by Steiner in detail.[1] As he indicated repeatedly, both in his general inquiries into human nature and in his pedagogical and medical lectures, the forces that build up the human body are the very same ones that later become available to us as mental powers. When the forces of development and growth have finished their work in the child's organism and are no longer needed there, they metamorphose into psycho-spiritual forces. Thus the forces of thought activity are the same as those that build up the human organism. Their laws are found in all of nature, and through thought activity itself we can recognize them as laws of nature. Human beings bear within themselves all the laws of nature. Our bodies and vital functions serves as visible knowledge—wisdom made manifest. Through a meditative dialog between our organism and our cognitive forces,

---

1   The path within is elaborated in detail by Steiner, particularly *Macrocosm and Microcosm* (CW 119). The difficulties and dangers encountered on this path are made quite clear in these lectures.

these spiritual principles can be experienced and made conscious once more. The human being comes into the world essentially knowing—knowing even the content of what we call science today; only this knowledge does not live in us consciously but is interwoven with our organism and our whole being. The human can be regarded as a microcosm, a synthesis of the macrocosm, and so within us we can find everything that exists outside of us in the world. In his widely noted book *The Tao of Physics*, Fritjof Capra demonstrated that Eastern knowledge acquired on the inner path bears an astonishing similarity to the picture of the world discovered and developed on the outer path by atomic physics.

A fact sometimes overlooked is that many of the discoveries of modern science were not made systematically on the outer path, but in part—in fact, in their crucial steps—on the inner path as well. A well-known and striking example is August Kekulé's discovery of the benzene ring.[2] For a long time he had been puzzled by the question of how the atoms in organic carbon compounds were arranged. It was on his way to a congress on a London omnibus that he reached his decisive insights. Dozing off on the horse-drawn vehicle, he dreamed of a great ball at the imperial court in Vienna. The men were dressed in old-fashioned dark suits, the women in light colors. Suddenly six dark-suited dancers formed a ring with the light-colored ones circling around it. At that moment Kekulé awoke and saw the solution to the arrangement of the atoms in carbon compounds: "I've got it! The answer is the ring!"

Characteristically, his initial experience of knowledge was couched in images and only later, when his waking consciousness returned, was it translated into an abstract formula. On the inner path, knowledge first appears in the form of images that must later be conceptually penetrated—abstracted—in the cognitive act.

---

2   Bernard Lievegoed cites this example in his book *Man on the Threshold*.
     Further examples of groundbreaking scientific discoveries made in a half-
     sleeping state are given by C. G. Jung in his book *Man and His Symbols*.

A Note on the History of Fairy Tales

Background of the Grimm Brothers' Fairy-Tale Collection[3]

The first impulses for a German fairy-tale collection came from significant literary figures in the Romantic movement—Achim von Arnim, Clemens Brentano, and Phillip Otto Runge. In 1807, Brentano visited the Grimm brothers in Kassel, where they were employed as librarians. He suggested that they collect fairy tales to be transcribed and prepared for publication.[4] As a model, he presented them with a copy of the two Runge tales, "The Fisherman and his Wife" and "The Juniper Tree." For the brothers, this suggestion was to lead to a central part of their life's work, culminating in the fairy-tale collection that has become, after the Bible, the most widely read book in German literature.

At the start of their work, the brothers used old manuscripts from the Kassel library. Only later, beginning in 1811, did they turn to oral sources. The first volume of the Grimms' fairy-tale collection, published in 1812, derives largely from written sources; the second, published three years later, contains mostly orally transmitted tales.

One of the most important sources for the orally transmitted tales was a tailor's wife of Huguenot ancestry named Dorothea Viehmann, now referred to as the *Märchenfrau* of Kassel. Once she had finished selling her wares at the Kassel marketplace, she would go to the Grimms' apartment for a cup of coffee and tell them fairy tales. Another source was Dorothea Wild, daughter of a pharmacist

---

3   Based primarily on three publications: 1) Hermann Grimm, *Household Stories by the Brothers Grimm*; 2) Karl Boegner, *Es war einmal—die Entstehung der Grimmschen Märchen* (Once Upon a Time: The Emergence of the Grimm Fairy Tale); 3) Heinz Rölleke, "Kinder- und Hausmärchen, gesammelt durch die Brüder Grimm." Transcriptions and commentaries by Heinz Rölleke.

4   The role played by the town of Kassel in the Rosicrucian stream has been revealed by Ludwig Klubert in his study "Where the first Rosicrucian texts were printed," published in the *Mitteilungen aus der anthroposophischen Arbeit in Deutschland*, no. 4, Christmas 1981.

from Bern who had settled in Kassel.[5] Sitting in the apothecary garden, the brothers heard from her tales such as "Hansel and Gretel," "The Wishing Table," "Mother Holle," "The Three Little Men in the Wood," "Allerleirauh" (All Kinds of Fur), "Sweetheart Roland," and "The Six Swans" (to be discussed in our study). Later, Dorothea Wild married Wilhelm Grimm. Besides "Dörtchen," as she was called, her six sisters and her mother also contributed tales, among them "Prince Swan," "Our Lady's Child," and "Simpleton."

The Wilds and Grimms were friends of a patrician family named Hassenpflug, in which the mother was of French stock. From her daughter Jeannette the Grimms learned many of the tales that went into the first volume. She is also the source for "Snow White," another of the tales that we shall examine later. The eldest of the Hassenpflug daughters was named Marie and has been identified by Rölleke as the storyteller indicated in the Grimms' note "from Marie." Hermann Grimm, son of Wilhelm Grimm, had mistakenly connected this note with the old Marie who lived in the Wild household as wet-nurse and nanny.

Other significant sources were the young women of the von Haxthausen and von Droste-Hülshoff families—in other words, nobility.[6] Thus as a rule the sources were not simple people of the "folk," but members of distinguished, often patrician families. Nor were they elderly; in fact, most were young and only a few middle-aged.

Originally the brothers had no thought at all of publishing on their own, but placed the first fruits of their collecting at the disposal of Clemens Brentano so that he could edit and publish them.

---

5   Steiner speaks of Dorothea Wild's character and her significance for the genesis of the fairy-tale collection in his lecture of Nov. 14, 1914, in the lecture course *Der Zusammenhang des Menschen mit der elementarischen Welt* (The Connection between Humankind and the Elemental World).

6   One of these was Annette von Droste-Hülshoff (1797–1848), whose mother was a von Haxthausen and who would later become a celebrated German poet (TN).

However, when this did not occur, the brothers were encouraged by Achim von Arnim to publish the tales themselves. He also found a publisher in Berlin for these still unknown and penniless librarians.

The manuscripts of the brothers Grimm have been lost, but the copy of the original version of the fairy-tale collection that was sent to Clemens Brentano was discovered in the Trappist Monastery Olenberg in the Alsace. Through it we can recognize how intensively the brothers Grimm worked on the fairy-tale material over time. From the first original version to the first book publication to the second edition and the following five editions published in the brothers' lifetime, crucial textual alterations were carried out. Each new edition was reworked and supplemented as various versions were brought together and their language stylized in such a way that the fairy tales might speak more directly to the soul. New tales were introduced and others removed. The style of the fairy tales was shaped by Wilhelm Grimm; it was he who created the Grimm genre. From this perspective Karl Boegner distinguishes between the Grimm brothers' tales and other literary fairy tales; they are "not subjective, not works of imaginative genius, as are those of Brentano and other authors, but 'objective fantasy'—recollections of experiences, harking intuitively back to the true skaldic tradition." According to Steiner, the Grimm brothers stood under higher spiritual guidance in their work.[7]

Fairy Tales as Rosicrucian Wisdom

Fairy-tale motifs derive in part from ancient mystery wisdom cultivated in the secret mystery centers of the Middle Ages—the temples of the Rosicrucian spiritual stream described by Steiner.[8] These centers disseminated their wisdom not in abstract teachings but through

---

7   Steiner, *Das Geheimnis des Todes. Wesen und Bedeutung Mitteleuropas und die europäischen Volksgeister* (The Secret of Death. The Nature and Meaning of Central Europe and the European Folk Spirits), May 15, 1915, Prague.

8   Steiner, *Background to the Gospel of St. Mark,* June 10, 1911, Berlin.

traveling storytellers.[9] From the mystery centers, these emissaries went from village to village spreading Rosicrucian wisdom in the form of fairy tales. People were receptive to the stories because they enjoyed listening to them. They were fired with the powerful imaginative life of these tales, and this enthusiasm helped impress the stories deeply in their souls. This in turn awakened the soul forces that would seek to understand these tales.

The time was not yet ripe for people to comprehend in a purely conceptual form the wisdom on which the tales were based. The tales first had to live as pictures in the soul, where they could become the germ of a future capacity to understand the spiritual relationships described imaginatively in them.

Fairy Tales Originating in the Folk Soul

Fairy tales with an origin of the kind just described have mixed with those from another source, out of which fairy tales have nourished the soul since time immemorial. For as long as there have been written records, fairy tales can be shown to have existed. In fact, one fairy-tale motif preserved on Egyptian papyri and stele completely parallels the story of "The Two Brothers" in the Grimms' collection. According to Steiner, the setting for this type of origin lies far in the past, when many human beings were still more or less clairvoyant.[10] Those who were able to retain such clairvoyance for a long time had experiences of the spiritual world in the state between sleeping and waking. They experienced it in the form of multifarious pictures. These experiences were not like the dreaming we experience at present, which is generally chaotic; rather, in this ancient clairvoyance the experiences were regular and occurred in many people in the same way.

---

9   The author, following Steiner's usage, speaks of them as "rhapsodists"—a term otherwise applied only to the traveling performers of epic poems in ancient Greece (TN).

10 Steiner, *Die Mission der neuen Geistesoffenbarung. Das Christus-Ereignis als Mittelpunktsgeschehen der Erdenevolution* (The Mission of the New Spiritual Revelation. The Christ Event as the Middle Point of Earth Evolution), Dec. 19, 1911, Berlin.

Thus in primeval times many people had such spiritual experiences in the form of pictorial clairvoyance. Receptivity to such perceptions grew ever less, however, until those who still had them put these soul-spiritual experiences into story form. In this way fairy tales arose and passed from place to place. In the process, they also spread through various languages, and so it happens that around the entire world similarities can be discerned in the body of fairy tales. Again, the source of these fairy tales does not lie only in hermetically guarded mystery wisdom; their origin is also to be found in the untutored "folk." Yet the two paths by which fairy tales entered the world have doubtless mixed, and it is quite possible that a tale can derive both from mystery wisdom as well as from the folk. Furthermore, fairy tales may well have developed further as they were improved and expanded by people who still possessed this natural spirituality, as was the case with the brothers Grimm.

Fairy Tales Themselves are Healing Remedies

Originally, the Grimm brothers intended their *Children's and Household Tales* for adults just as much as for children. They saw in these tales something akin to Greek mythology. But as it happened, the adults found it difficult to relate to fairy tales, and so they became the province of children—at least initially.

There are the most varied approaches to interpreting fairy tales; each offers a mirror to a particular worldview in which to see itself. Hence individuals each experience fairy tales differently and will understand them in accordance with their own worldview. From completely different points of view than Steiner's, both Sigmund Freud and C. G. Jung cast light on the importance of fairy tales for adults. Since then the Jungian psychotherapists in particular have embraced the fairy tale. They explain its significance by viewing fairy-tale motifs as the purest and simplest expression of the collective unconscious. From this point of view, fairy tales reflect archetypal patterns of the soul. Their motifs represent our psychological self in pictures, as it were, so that we can recognize ourselves in them. Therefore in psychotherapy, the processes of reaching self-knowledge and finding one's self can be initiated by practicing an intensive inner experience of the fairy-tale motifs.

Although Jungian psychotherapy explains the fairy tales purely psychologically and does not include a comprehensive understanding of man and the world like the anthroposophic interpretations, its judgment about the significance of fairy tales is similar to Steiner's; fairy tales have a healing effect; they are a kind of spiritual medicine; they heal through their spiritual content. In fact, they are "medicine" in the truest sense of the word.

Outer-World Imaginations as Mirrors of the Inner World

In fairy tales, processes within the human being are always depicted in images. The imaginative world can embrace the full complexity and multi-dimensionality of any issue in life, especially in our inner life. Various aspects of one particular issue—which we will see as various aspects of a particular planetary metal sphere—are imagined through different characters or creatures in the fairy tale. Each person in the fairy tale, with his specific character and behavior, represents a different aspect of the diverse forces of a certain planetary sphere. Thus the outer world portrayed in the fairy tale mirrors different aspects of our inner world, including the opposite efforts often at work in our soul, which all originate from the same metal sphere. The evidence for this is found in the correspondences we shall reveal between fairy-tale images and remedy action.

The Grimms' Fairy Tales as Musical Compositions

Steiner pointed repeatedly to the spiritual aspect of fairy tales, showing how their composition corresponds to spiritual laws. In them live both the spirituality of the human being and the spiritual of the world. Therefore the fairy tales contain mysteries in imaginative form—mysteries not only of the earthly world and humankind, but also of the cosmos. This explains why our study is able to consider not only inner-human but also cosmological processes and can speak of the action of the planetary spheres on man. This is the special perspective of the fairy tales.

Because of these connections, the effect of fairy tales on the human soul is a primal and elemental one. In a certain way it can be compared to that of classical music. Both music and fairy tales bring the soul of the listener into sympathetic motion and can evoke the deepest feelings. In a musical composition there is a particular mood, associated with its key, and motifs that are repeated in variations. Similarly, in each of the fairy tales considered here we encounter a very particular mood, comparable to the musical key, and a motif that runs through the plot in various metamorphoses. The mood and the variations of the motif are what draw us in and bring our soul into resonance. The effect of fairy tales goes further than this, however. The sequence of pictures—the imaginative content of the tale—enables us as readers or listeners to identify with particular characters or figures. We recognize ourselves. Yet we experience ourselves not as we would like to see ourselves or as we believe ourselves to be, but in a way that corresponds to the structure of our soul. In this way we can become aware of fundamental conflicts in our soul; in other words, the fairy tale can initiate a process of self-recognition. Yet this mirror of the self not only allows us to recognize conflicts and weaknesses; it also points the way to overcoming them. By inwardly working through those fairy tales that embody a relevant set of issues, we become acquainted with our own possibilities for spiritual growth. This is always a healing process, since it opens the path to finding ourselves. In Jungian language this path is known as individuation; in anthroposophy it is called the process of initiation. On this path, the fairy tale can be of critical help.

Thus the deep effects of fairy tales come about through two elements—soul resonance and cognitive identification. Together, the two are able to produce the special effect that fairy tales can have.

Together, they evoke the sense of personal affectedness we experience when we work with a relevant fairy tale—the feeling of being touched not only in mind and soul, but even on the physiological level. In particular therapeutic situations, a fairy tale can cause malaise, nausea, dizziness and similar symptoms. Such a comprehensive action is what gives the fairy tale true remedy character. Thus it should not be surprising that anthroposophic clinics hold fairy-tale evenings for their patients, or that psychotherapists and psychiatrists engage in fairy-tale study.[11]

A statement by Steiner gives a sense for how deeply fairy tales act in the unconscious: "What the human being experiences as aesthetic enjoyment of a fairy tale is certainly very far removed from what goes on in the unconscious depths of the human soul, from what unites with the human soul, because the soul has an ineradicable need—just as the organism has a need—for nutrients, for nourishment to flow through it."[12]

11 Christa-Johanna Bub, "Warum gestalten wir Märchenabende für unsere Patienten?," 20. Rundbrief des Carl Gustav Carus Institutes und der Klinik Öschelbronn, 1986–1987. Gerhard Kienle, "Zur künstlerischen und gruppenpädagogischen Behandlung der Pubertätskrisen," *Zeitschrift für Psychotherapie und medizinische Psychologie,* no. 2, pp. 70–77, March 1960. Gerhard Kienle, Das Märchen in der Psychotherapie," *Zeitschrift für Psychotherapie und medizinische Psychologie,* no. 2, pp. 47–53, 1959.

12 Steiner, *Ergebnisse der Geistesforschung* (The Results of Spiritual Research), Feb. 6, 1913, Berlin.

PLANETARY SPHERES, METALS, CHARACTER AND PHYSIOLOGY

The Planetary Spheres

The use of metals as remedies is based on the recognition that they stand in a cosmological connection with certain organs and processes in the human body.[1] This cosmological connection is based on a relationship of the metals to particular planets. What acts upon the metals is not, of course, the planets as we see them in the sky, but the planetary spheres. The planet visible to the eye is merely the localized physical embodiment of its sphere, which extends far beyond the planet itself, embracing its entire orbit. Acting within this sphere are high spiritual beings whose forces were at work in the creation of the metals on Earth. Their forces are also active in particular organs and processes in the human being. Hence there is an inner relationship between planet, metal and organ or organ process—a relationship that was known in ancient times and has been revealed again by Rudolf Steiner in a form suited to our modern consciousness. The following connections exist:

---

1   The relationship between planets, metals, and organs is described repeatedly from different perspectives in the work of Steiner. Particular presentations are cited in the following chapters in connection with the individual metals and illnesses. Here we will simply point to Steiner's lectures to the workers at the Goetheanum, *From Comets to Cocaine...* (Feb. 10, 1923, Dornach).

PLANET	METAL	ORGAN
Saturn	Lead	Spleen
Jupiter	Tin	Liver
Mars	Iron	Gallbladder
Sun	Gold	Heart
Venus	Copper	Kidneys
Mercury	Mercury	Lungs
Moon	Silver	Brain

Relics of the once-known connection between metal and planet are found in names such as *Mercury,* referring both to the metal and to the corresponding planet, or in terms such as *saturnism,* which refers to lead poisoning.

The initiates of times past who experienced the connections between planets, metal and organs expressed them in a verse of sacred wisdom, which according to Steiner had something like the following form:

> Being born of the cosmos, oh you in form of light,
> Empowered by the Sun in the might of the Moon—
>
> You are gifted with Mars' creative sounding
> And Mercury's limb-moving oscillation,
>
> You are illumined by Jupiter's radiant wisdom
> And Venus' love-bearing beauty.
> May Saturn's age-old spirit-inwardness
> Consecrate you to being-in-space and becoming-in-time!

Touching on each planet, the verse expresses how it acts in its characteristic way on the human being.[2] These motifs will be our

---

2   Of interest in this connection is a verse ascribed to Basilius Valentinus, which also shows a living knowledge of the "being nature" of the planetary spheres: "Oh Sun, King of this world/Luna sustains your race/Mercury couples you/Without Venus's favor you achieve

focus in the following chapters on the fairy tales. First, however, we need to consider how the planetary forces affect the prenatal existence of individual human beings.

The Planetary Spheres and the Path to Incarnation

Let us look more closely at the connection between planet, organ, and human character. Forces emanating from the planets are not only responsible for the materialization of the metals on Earth; they also have their role in the inception of each human existence. On its path to earthly incarnation, the human "I" experiences each of the planetary spheres in succession. Setting out on this path, it first experiences the Saturn sphere, the portal to the planetary realm of the Earth. In connecting itself with the being of the Saturn sphere, the "I" takes in specific principles underlying organ formation and organ processes. At the same time it receives dispositions for certain soul qualities. Once this has occurred, the "I" enters the Jupiter sphere and is imbued with its qualities while further organ processes and soul predispositions are taken in. Next it passes through the Mars sphere and joins with its forces. And in like manner it passes on through the Sun, Venus, Mercury, and Moon spheres before reaching the Earth, where it unites with a specific hereditary stream.

Thus in its progression through the planetary spheres toward the Earth, the "I" takes in the characteristic qualities of each. As a whole, these qualities compose the star, or astral, body.[3] Yet each individuality unites with the planetary spheres differently and in this way receives a disposition that suits the requirements of its karmic development. According to what the individuality brings with

nothing/Whoever has chosen Mars as husband/Never loses Jove's favor/So that Saturn old and hoary/May show himself in many colors."
Steiner discusses this verse in *The Riddle of Man*, Sept. 3 1916, Dornach.

3   The incarnation path is described variously by Steiner in lectures. One aspect is presented here. On Dec. 18, 1921, he explained that the astral body is informed by its experience of solar movement—in the powers of thinking, feeling, and willing we experience an image of solar movements (*Mystery of the Universe*).

it out of previous Earth lives, it receives the soul motifs with which it will have to deal in its earthly destiny. Once the "I" has traversed the entire path from the Saturn sphere to the Moon sphere, its new astral body has been formed for the coming incarnation. The individual's character traits have now taken form, with all of their possibilities and longings, their strengths and weaknesses.

An awareness of this background is essential for an understanding of the presentations to follow. Each of the seven fairy tales has quite a particular mood, through which we are able to describe the corresponding metal in its relation to the human being. The mood is an expression of the essential nature of the given planetary sphere and hence also of the psychic and organic traits predisposed there. And since the motifs of the fairy tale also possess connections with the planetary spheres, they also help us understand the process-aspect of the metals. In summary it can be said that the mood and motifs of a tale point to a planetary sphere, to a certain metal and metal process-action in the human being, as well as to a corresponding soul disposition.

The Planetary Metals as Orchestrators
of Signaling Pathways in the Organism

With the exception of iron and copper, little or no trace of the other planetary metals is found in the human organism. How is it then that these metals play such an important role in the organism as we indicate in this study? The planetary metal spheres act like conductors of an orchestra, forging up to fifty instrumentalists into a harmonious whole. What we hear are the instruments. We are not necessarily aware of a conductor simply from hearing the music. Indeed, all that we see of conductors during a performance is their back, and yet they play a literally central role in orchestrating the various instrumentalists. The metallic planetary spheres act in a similar way. They orchestrate the various pathways connected with their sphere. The Saturn or lead sphere orchestrates the various signaling pathways of the lipid metabolism, generating warmth in the organism. In the warmth of our organism, the Ancient Saturn sphere is still present in us today. In a similar way the planetary Moon or silver sphere orchestrates the signaling pathways of the sugar metabolism. Energy metabolism, neurological functions and reproductive processes are connected with the sugar metabolism, all of which is coordinated by the silver sphere in us. The details of these aspects will be described in the interpretations of the corresponding fairy tales.

The Seven Main Metals as Remedies in the Mirror of the Fairy Tales

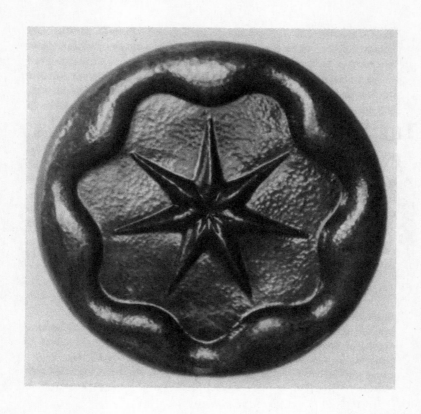

Saturn Seal

LEAD AS A REMEDY: "FAITHFUL JOHN"

There was, once upon a time, an old king who was ill and thought to himself, "I am lying on what must be my deathbed." Then he said, "Tell Faithful John to come to me." Faithful John was his favorite servant, and was so called, because he had for his whole life long been so true to him. When therefore he came beside the bed, the King said to him, "Most faithful John, I feel my end approaching and have no anxiety except about my son. He is still of tender age and cannot always know how to guide himself. If you do not promise me to teach him everything that he ought to know, and to be his foster-father, I cannot close my eyes in peace."

Then Faithful John answered, "I will not forsake him and will serve him with fidelity, even if it should cost me my life." On this, the old King said, "Now I die in comfort and peace." Then he added, "After my death, you shall show him the whole castle—all the chambers, halls, and vaults, and all the treasures therein, but the last chamber in the long gallery, in which is the picture of the princess of the Golden Dwelling, you shall not show. If he sees that picture, he will fall violently in love with her, and will drop down in a swoon, and go through great danger for her sake; therefore you must preserve him from that." And when Faithful John had once more given his promise to the old King about this, the King said no more, but laid his head on his pillow and died.

When the old King had been carried to his grave, Faithful John told the young King all that he had promised his father on his deathbed and said, "This will I assuredly perform and will be faithful to you as I have been faithful to him, even if it should cost me my life."

When the mourning was over, Faithful John said to him, "It is now time that you should see your inheritance. I will show you your father's palace." Then he took him about everywhere, up and down, and let him see all the riches, and the magnificent apartments, only there was one room which he did not open, that in which hung the dangerous picture. The picture was, however, so placed that when the door was opened you looked straight on it, and it was so admirably painted that it seemed to breathe and live, and there was nothing more charming or more beautiful in the whole world.

The young King, however, plainly remarked that Faithful John always walked past this one door and said, "Why do you never open this one for me?"

"There is something within it," he replied, "that would terrify you."

However, the King answered, "I have seen all the palace, and I will know what is in this room also," and he went and tried to break open the door by force.

Then Faithful John held him back and said, "I promised your father before his death that you should not see what is in this chamber, it might bring the greatest misfortune on you and on me."

"Ah, no," replied the young King, "if I do not go in, it will be my certain destruction. I should have no rest day or night until I had seen it with my own eyes. I shall not leave the place now until you have unlocked the door."

Faithful John saw that there was no help for it now and, with a heavy heart and many sighs, sought out the key from the great bunch. When he had opened the door, he went in first and thought by standing before him he could hide the portrait so that the King should not see it in front of him, but what availed that? The King stood on tiptoe and saw it over his shoulder. And when he saw the portrait of the maiden, which was so magnificent and shone with gold and precious stones, he fell fainting to the ground. Faithful John took him up, carried him to his bed, and sorrowfully thought, "The misfortune has befallen us, Lord God, what will be the end of it?"

Then he strengthened him with wine until he came to himself again. The first words the King said were, "Ah, the beautiful portrait! Whose is it?"

"That is the princess of the Golden Dwelling," Faithful John answered.

Then the King continued, "My love for her is so great, that if all the leaves on all the trees were tongues, they could not declare it. I will give my life to win her. You are my most Faithful John, you must help me."

The faithful servant considered within himself for a long time how to set about the matter, for it was difficult even to obtain a sight of the King's daughter. At length he thought of a way and said to the King, "Everything which she has about her is of gold—tables, chairs, dishes, glasses, bowls, and household furniture. Among your treasures are five tons of gold; let one of the goldsmiths of the Kingdom work these up into all manner of vessels and utensils, into all kinds of birds, wild beasts and strange animals, such as may please her, and we will go there with them and try our luck."

The King ordered all the goldsmiths to be brought to him, and they had to work night and day until at last the most splendid things were prepared. When everything was stowed on board a ship, Faithful John put on the dress of a merchant, and the King was forced to do the same to make himself quite unrecognizable. Then they sailed across the sea and sailed on until they came to the town wherein dwelled the princess of the Golden Dwelling.

Faithful John asked the King to remain behind on the ship and wait for him. "Perhaps I shall bring the princess with me," he said. "Therefore, see that everything is in order; have the golden vessels set out and the whole ship decorated." Then he gathered in his apron all kinds of gold things, went to shore and walked straight to the royal palace.

When he entered the palace courtyard, a beautiful girl was standing by the well with two golden buckets in her hand and drawing water with them. As she was turning to carry away the sparkling water, she saw the stranger and asked who he was. He answered, "I am a merchant," and opened his apron, and let her look in.

She cried, "Oh, what beautiful gold things!" She set down her pails and looked at the golden wares one after the other. The girl said, "The princess must see these; she has such great pleasure in golden things that she will buy all you have." She took him by the hand and led him upstairs, for she was the waiting-maid.

When the King's daughter saw the wares, she was quite delighted and said, "They are so beautifully worked, that I will buy them all of you."

Faithful John said, "I am only the servant of a rich merchant. The things I have here cannot be compared to those my master has on his ship. They are the most beautiful and valuable things that have ever been made in gold." She wanted to have everything brought to her, but he said, "There are so many of them that it would take a great many days to do that, and so many rooms would be required to exhibit them that your house is not big enough."

Her curiosity and longing became even more excited until, at last, she said, "Conduct me to the ship. I will go there myself and behold the treasures of your master."

On this Faithful John was quite delighted and led her to the ship, and when the King saw her, he perceived that her beauty was even greater than the picture had represented it to be, and thought no other than that his heart would burst in twain. Then she got into the ship, and the King led her within. Faithful John, however, remained behind with the pilot and ordered the ship to be pushed off, saying, "Set all sail, till it fly like a bird in air." Within, however, the King showed her the golden vessels, every one of them, also the wild beasts and strange animals.

Many hours went by while she was seeing everything, and in her delight she did not observe that the ship was sailing away. After she had looked at the last, she thanked the merchant and wanted to go home, but when she came to the side of the ship, she saw that it was on the deep sea far from land and hurrying onward with all sail set. "Ah," cried she in her alarm, "I am betrayed! I am carried away and have fallen into the power of a merchant—I would die rather!"

The King, however, seized her hand and said, "I am not a merchant. I am a king and of no meaner origin than you are, and if I have carried you away with subtlety, that has come to pass because of my exceeding great love for you. The first time that I looked on your portrait, I fell fainting to the ground." When the princess of the Golden Dwelling heard that, she was comforted, and her heart was inclined unto him, so that she willingly consented to be his wife.

It so happened, however, while they were sailing onward over the deep sea, that Faithful John, who was sitting on the fore part of the vessel, making music, saw three ravens in the air, which came flying toward them. With this, he stopped playing and listened to what they were saying to each other, which he well understood. One cried, "Oh, there he is carrying home the princess of the Golden Dwelling."

"Yes," replied the second, "but he has not got her yet."

"But he has got her, she is sitting beside him in the ship," said the third.

Then the first began again and cried, "What good will that do him? When they reach land, a chestnut horse will leap forth to meet him, and the prince will wish to mount it. But if he does that, it will run away with him and rise into the air, and he will never again see his maiden."

"But is there no escape?" said the second.

"Oh, yes, if anyone else gets on it swiftly, takes out the pistol that must be in its holster, and shoots the horse dead with it, the young King is saved. But who knows that? And whoever does know it, and tells it to him will be turned to stone from the toe to the knee."

Then the second said, "I know more than that; even if the horse be killed, the young King will still not keep his bride. When they go into the castle together, a wrought bridal garment will be lying there in a dish, and looking as if it were woven of gold and silver; it is, however, nothing but sulfur and pitch, and if he put it on, it will burn him to the very bone and marrow."

"Is there no escape at all?" said the third.

"Oh, yes," replied the second, "if anyone wearing gloves seizes the garment and throws it into the fire and burns it, the young King will be saved.

"But what avails that?"

"Whoever knows it and tells it to him, half his body will become stone from the knee to the heart."

Then the third said, "I know yet more. Even if the bridal garment be burned, the young king will still not have his bride. After the wedding, when the dancing begins and the young queen is dancing, she will suddenly turn pale and fall as if dead, and if someone does not lift her and draw three drops of blood from her right breast and spit them out again, she will die. But if anyone who knows and were to declare it, that one would become stone from the crown of the head to the sole of the foot."

When the ravens had spoken of this together, they flew on, and Faithful John had understood everything well. But from that time forth, he became quiet and sad, for if he concealed what he had heard from his master, the latter would be unfortunate, and if he revealed it to him, he himself must sacrifice his life. Finally, however, he said to himself, "I will save my master, even if it destroys me."

When they came ashore, all happened as foretold by the ravens, and a magnificent chestnut horse sprang forth. "Good," said the King, "he shall carry me to my palace." He was about to mount it when Faithful John stood before him, jumped quickly upon it, drew the pistol out of the holster, and shot the horse.

The other attendants of the King, who were not, after all, very fond of Faithful John, cried, "How shameful to kill the beautiful animal that was about to carry the King to his palace."

But the King said, "Hold your peace and leave him alone; he is my most faithful John. He knows what may be the good of that!"

They entered the palace and, in the hall, stood a dish and therein the bridal garment, looking as if made of gold and silver. The young king approached it and was about to take hold of it, but Faithful John pushed him away, seized it with gloves, carried it quickly to the fire and burned it. The other attendants again began to murmur and said, "Behold, now he is even burning the King's bridal garment!"

The young king said, however, "Who knows what good he may have done; leave him be. He is my most faithful John."

Now the wedding was solemnized; the dance began, and the bride also took part in it. Faithful John was alert and looked into her face. Suddenly she turned pale and fell to the ground as if dead. With this, he hastily ran to her, lifted her, and bore her into a chamber. He laid her down, knelt, sucked the three drops of blood from her right breast, and spat them out. Immediately she breathed again and recovered, but the young king had seen this, and being ignorant why Faithful John had done it was angry and cried, "Throw him into a dungeon."

Next morning, Faithful John was condemned and led to the gallows. When he stood on high and was about to be executed, he said, "Everyone who has to die is permitted before the end to make one last speech; may I, too, claim the right?"

"Yes," answered the King, "it shall be granted to you."

Then Faithful John said, "I am unjustly condemned and have always been true to you." He then related how he had listened to the ravens' conversation while on the sea and how he had been obliged to do all these things to save his master.

Then the King cried, "Oh, my most Faithful John, pardon, pardon—bring him down." However, as Faithful John spoke the last word, he fell lifeless and became a stone.

With this, the King and the Queen suffered great anguish, and the King said, "Ah, how ill I have repaid great fidelity!" He ordered the stone figure to be carried up and placed in his bedroom beside his bed. As often as he looked on it, he wept and said, "Ah, if I could bring you to life again, my most faithful John."

Time passed and the Queen bore twins, two sons who grew fast and were her delight. Once when the Queen was at church and the two children sat playing beside their father, who, full of grief, again looked at the stone figure, sighed, and said, "Ah, if I could only bring you to life again, my most faithful John."

Then the stone began to speak and said, "You can bring me to life again if you will use what is dearest to you for that purpose."

Then the King cried, "I will give everything I have in the world for you."

The stone continued, "If you will cut off the heads of your two children with your own hand and sprinkle me with their blood, I will be restored to life."

The King was terrified when he heard that he himself must kill his dearest children, but he thought of faithful John's great fidelity and how he had died for him. He drew his sword and with his own hand cut off the children's heads. When he had smeared the stone with their blood, life returned to it, and Faithful John stood once more safe and healthy before him.

He said to the King, "Your truth shall not go unrewarded."

He took the children's heads, put them on again, and rubbed the wounds with their blood. Immediately, they became whole again and jumped about and went on playing as if nothing had happened. The King was full of joy, and when he saw the Queen coming he hid Faithful John and the two children in a great cupboard. When she entered, he said to her, "Have you been praying in the church?"

"Yes," she answered, "but I have been thinking constantly of Faithful John and what misfortune befell him through us."

Then he said, "Dear wife, we can give him his life again, but it will cost us our two little sons, whom we must sacrifice." The Queen turned pale and her heart was full of terror, but she said, "We owe it to him, for his great fidelity."

Then the King rejoiced that she thought as he had. He went and opened the cupboard and brought forth Faithful John and the children. He said, "God be praised, he is delivered, and we have our little sons again as well," and told her how everything had occurred. Then they lived together in great happiness until their death.[1]

～

The tale of "Faithful John" belongs at the beginning of our discussion since it casts a differentiated light on the lead process, the first metal dynamic encountered by the individuality on its path to incarnation.

The lead forces are connected with the planet Saturn, and the lead process for an earthly life is prepared when the "I" enters the planetary sphere of Saturn. Seen from the point of view of the "I" on its incarnation path, this sphere forms the portal and outermost boundary of our planetary system.

Before turning to the fairy tale let us describe the properties of lead itself and attempt to experience qualities that we can assign imaginatively to the lead sphere and then illustrate through the fairy tale.

Characteristic Qualities of Lead

When we contemplate a piece of lead, the dark-gray metal strikes us as heavy and cold. When we take it into our hand, the heaviness is confirmed but not the coldness—in fact it feels surprisingly soft and warm. Let us look at the phenomenological aspects that help explain this.

Lead does not conduct heat like other metals, but seems to "swallow" it and store it within. When heated, lead expands considerably, as if swelling from the accumulated heat. This inner warmth is a characteristic of lead that we shall encounter repeatedly in our discussion.

Lead brings almost all outer influences to a standstill, hence its obstructing, retarding influence even on impacts of tremendous force. Lead absorbs mechanical vibrations, which is why it is used in testing explosives. This is done using a cube of lead with a cylindrical cavity extending mid-way down within it. When an explosion is set off in

---

1   Trans. by Margaret Taylor (1884); from http://classiclit.about.com/library /bl-etexts/grimm/bl-grimm-faithful.htm.

this, a form alteration of greater or lesser extent results, but no further damage. The violence of the explosion is stifled in the sluggish metal. Every outer impact leaves an impression in lead that is retained to an extent. Spatial movement comes to a stop in lead. This quality also accounts for lead's delimiting and shielding action. Lead paint protects metals from rusting. It is used when a high degree of insulation is desired, for example in coffins. Lead aprons protect from exposure to radiation. Certain corrosive chemicals, such as sulfuric acid and hydrofluoric acid, can be safely stored in lead containers.

Another important property of lead in this connection is its inner luminosity. In various compounds lead manifests this quality in creating shiny paints with good covering properties.

Finally, in terms of its mood connotation, the word *leaden* applies to situations in which time seems to have come to stop, as though frozen—when we experience it as oppressive. In such moments it is as though depression has set in; everything has weight; everything seems in the clutches of death.

Correspondence between the Fairy Tale and the Lead Process

The particular characteristics of lead, which can be summarized as forces of past-orientation, persistence, and rigidity, as well as warmth and inner luminosity, all reappear in the tale of "Faithful John" as human traits, deeds, and sufferings. Warmth becomes self-sacrifice; persistence and past-orientation become loyalty; heaviness and rigidity become the willingness or even the longing for death; and inner luminosity becomes the power of resurrection. And these very traits of loyalty, self-sacrifice, rigidity, death and resurrection are the motifs out of which the plot of this tale is woven. John's loyalty is revealed to us in stark images; he takes devotion and dutifulness so far as to sacrifice his own life to save that of his king and master. And significantly, his death takes the form of the ultimate rigidity; he is turned to a stone figure.

Such images can be interpreted as imaginations of the Saturn, or lead, process, which Bernard Lievegoed describes as one of immobilization in spatial death.[2] The lead process leads to mineral-ization in the human organism, which reaches its death point in the skeleton. Yet the death point is not the endpoint. Bone is the birth-place of the second Saturn process; in the blood-forming activity of the bone marrow the lead process becomes a force of revitalization and resurrection. This too appears in the images of the fairy tale in the resurrection of John, which is made possible by a blood sacrifice. Nor is it confined to the servant; the king, too, feels bound in loy-alty to his servant. To bring him to life again, he sacrifices his own children and smears the petrified John with their blood. By virtue of their blood, John awakens from his petrified state rejuvenated and stronger than before.

It will be useful to look more closely at the quality of loyalty. It is rooted in three soul qualities that Rudolf Steiner describes as essence-characteristics of Saturn—inwardness, depth of soul, and memory.[3] For loyalty to exist the past must remain permanently etched in the memory; it must mature there and deepen the mind. The present, in contrast, touches us less. This insight enables us to understand the actions of the servant and the king. Rudolf Steiner describes the being of Saturn as follows: "Altogether, Saturn is the cosmic body in our planetary system that gives itself utterly in its own being; and its essence is gradually revealed as a kind of memory of our solar system, and it speaks of the past of the solar system with inner warmth and with fervor. It is what eternally seduces us, as it were, to disregard the earthly."[4] When we take this description as a soul mood, we have little difficulty in finding its parallel in the char-acter of Faithful John. Thus we can say that "Faithful John," both in its central motifs and in its mood, reflects characteristic aspects of the being of Saturn and of the lead process. Now that we have

2   Lievegoed, *Man on the Threshold.*

3   Steiner, *Eurythmy as Visible Speech,* July 7, 1924, Dornach.

4   Steiner, *Initiationswissenschaft und Sternenerkenntnis* (Initiation Science and the Knowledge of the Stars).

considered the chief motifs of the tale, let us make a more detailed examination of its particular images.

The Lead Process in Its Various Aspects, as Shown in Specific Fairy-tale Images: The Lead Process and Memory

The opening image of the tale is that of a dying king. Before his death, the king bids his loyal servant John faithfully serve his son and successor and gives him an additional admonition—to "show him the whole castle—all the chambers, halls, and vaults, and all the treasures therein; but the last chamber in the long gallery, in which is the picture of the princess of the Golden Dwelling, you shall not show. If he sees that picture, he will fall violently in love with her and will drop down a swoon and go through great danger for her sake. Therefore, you must preserve him from that." After the old king's death, Faithful John shows the young king the entire castle, except for the forbidden room. Noticing this, the young king insists on seeing this room as well. With a heavy heart the servant unlocks the door, and the very thing that the old king had predicted before his death comes to pass: When the young king's eyes fall upon the image of the maiden, the Princess of the Golden Dwelling, he falls in a faint.

Let us approach this scenario by viewing the various elements of the plot in relation to the lead/Saturn process. The young king, in this context, can be interpreted as the "I" as it comes from the reaches of the cosmos to begin its path toward earthly incarnation. His entry into the forbidden chamber indicates that he has taken a decisive step into a new sphere—from our point of view, the planetary sphere of Saturn or lead. With this step the "I" begins its path toward incarnation, and so begin the adventures and dangers of becoming and being human. The young king enters the lead sphere unprepared and when he sees the portrait of the Princess of the Golden Dwelling, he is overwhelmed by its sensory impact and faints.

To understand this we must bring to mind the function of the lead process in the human being. It is only by incorporating the lead process that the human being first gains consciousness. Through it the vitality of sensory impressions is damped down to the point where they are no longer overwhelming.[5] This is what makes memory possible; for only when the sense impressions have been deadened and fixed can memory arise. With the prince's entry to the Saturn sphere—the room where the image of the Princess of the Golden Dwelling hangs—two overlapping processes happen. He is overwhelmed by the sensory impressions because he is still untouched by the lead forces; and at the same time he takes these forces in and they are able to begin acting within him. This is why the overpowering sense impression does not dissipate when he faints, but fixes itself in his memory. When the young prince awakens from his faint we can see that he has internalized the lead process and received the power of memory: "The beautiful portrait," he exclaims, "Whose is it?" "That is the Princess of the Golden Dwelling," answers Faithful John. "My love for her is so great, that if all the leaves on all the trees were tongues, they could not declare it. I will give my life to win her. You are my most Faithful John, you must help me." These words show how deeply the image of the princess has impressed itself on his soul. The faculty of memory has assumed its place and the image he perceived now lives there indelibly.

When the individuality enters the Saturn sphere, it sees the midpoint of this sphere, the luminous Sun. The Golden Dwelling is this Sun sphere, and the Princess of the Golden Dwelling, who surrounds herself with all the treasures of gold to be gotten, represents Sun-nature. For gold has always been seen as the metal and the symbol of the Sun.

The Lead Process and the Lost Light: Mystical excursus

To understand the Princess and her close connection to Saturn, we must make an *excursus* into the teachings of Jakob Böhme, who gained an intimate knowledge of the being she represents and

---

5   Steiner, *Mystery Knowledge and Mystery Centres*, Dec. 14, 1923, Dornach.

described it repeatedly. We must also be acquainted with the picture of cosmic and earthly evolution presented by Rudolf Steiner. The development of the world falls into seven great stages of planetary development or consciousness, of which our present physical-mineral Earth is the fourth. In the first of these stages, known as "Saturn" (and not to be confused with the planet of the same name), time arose; previously, timelessness had reigned. This "Saturn" was surrounded by the cosmic light forces of the zodiac but had no inner light of its own. Those initiated into these mysteries—among them Böhme—have referred to the essence of these light- and wisdom-filled cosmic forces under the image of the divine virgin, Sophia. The original human being—as yet a divine being before any fall—was in complete harmony with the being of Sophia. From this perspective she appears as a God figure, the sculptor of the divine image in man. She is the archetype that reveals God in the human and the human in God. Thus the theological world of Böhme comprises a divine fourfold quality: Father, Son, Spirit, and Sophia. Sophia is the fourth principle and the body of the triune divinity.

The period of ancient Saturn commenced when this harmony was abruptly shattered.[6] Primeval humankind abandoned the oneness of God because it did not offer him sufficient stimulation. People turned away from the divine Sophia to experience their self and the multiplicity of things. In this way humankind lost the condition of divinely illumined oneness and traded the all-embracing love of Sophia for the torments of doubt, polarity, and strife. Thus, people enter isolation, feel abandoned, and have intimations of death. Now that the divine Sophia no longer stands before us and all has become dark within, we have become aware of our impermanence. Time begins.

Thus begins the age that we are speaking of, the ancient Saturn condition, whose darkness and ominous atmosphere clearly remind us of this fall. Böhme refers to this primeval separation as the "first

---

6   On the "planetary stages" of cosmic evolution, see, for example, Steiner, *An Outline of Esoteric Science*, ch. 4.

fall." The fall depicted in the Bible would accordingly be a second, much later stage.

Deep in the being of Saturn, however, strongly lived an intuitive yearning-filled memory of the divine Light Maiden Sophia. Thus it makes sense to interpret the figure of the Princess of the Golden Dwelling (i.e., the world) as the Light Maiden, who is the divine Sophia or divine wisdom.[7] This interpretation also explains why the king's son is filled with such longing when he sees her image, and why he cannot go on living unless he succeeds in possessing her; it is longing for a lost unity that he must regain at all costs. Hence nothing can keep him from going in search of the Princess of the Golden Dwelling.

The Lead Process and Balancing
Rhythm-giving Forces in the Metabolic Area

In spite of the serious tone of this tale, there are episodes that have something amusing about them, as when the king's son and Faithful John go on their quest for the Princess disguised as merchants. It seems odd that figures whom we understand as personifications of the lead process would adopt the role of merchants. Merchants, after all, have always been associated with the god Mercury (Hermes), so that the king (and his servant) is assuming Mercury's role. Outwardly this appears to be an appreciable comedown from Kingship. How shall we understand it?

To respond, we must look into the connection between Saturn and Mercury. As Jung has pointed out, alchemical traditions were aware of an intimate kinship between these two planetary beings.[8] According to them, Mercury and Saturn share an identity, the difference being that "as Mercury he is *juvenis,* as Saturn *senex.*"[9] An

---

7   Schult, *Maria Sophia. Das ewig Weibliche in Gott, Mensch und Kosmos;* and Meyer, *The Wisdom of Fairy Tales.*

8   Jung, "Der Geist Mercurius," in *Psychologische Abhandlungen,* vol. 6, Rascher Verlag, Zurich, 1948.

9   Latin *juvenis* = young; *senex* = old. The quote is from Jung's *Alchemical Studies,* p. 250 (TN).

indication by Rudolf Steiner on the function of the spleen as a Sun organ casts light on this cryptic statement.

Steiner describes the critical role in food absorption played by the spleen, which mediates between the rhythms inherent in foods and the inner rhythms of the organism. The action of the spleen protects the organism from being overwhelmed by foreign influences. When overwhelmed, the human organism develops an allergic reaction such as a food allergy. Thus the spleen exercises a mediating activity between the inner and outer world (to which the foods belong). Mediating functions are Mercurial functions, and thus we can see how Saturn incorporates essential aspects of Mercury.

In regard to spleen activity we must be aware that as a Saturn organ the spleen has other functional dimensions. The aspect mentioned here falls in the domain of its etheric functions. Below we will meet another task of the spleen, having to do with the capacity for enthusiasm.

From this point of view, when the King and his servant take on a Mercurial role as personified Saturn processes, we can now understand it as a reference to the mediating, rhythm-creating lead forces. Through them the Saturn process can connect itself with the outer world, and foreign substance can be taken into the bodily self. Much as the sense organs perceive otherness and allow us to take it into our consciousness, the overall function of the spleen is an integrating one. The more a person's metabolic realm is permeated with individuality, the more pronounced is the lead process (which is connected with the Saturn organ of the spleen).

Let us continue with the fairy tale. Once the Princess has been tricked in this way—she does not even notice it when she is abducted from her homeland—the young king can dispense with his Mercury role and manifest his true nature. For this reason the Princess gives her assent to their alliance. But until the final union the real dangers associated with the Saturn sphere or lead process remain to be faced.

The Lead Process and Thinking

The dangers of the lead process are its deviations to one side or the other, and it is these that are now presented to us by the fairy tale in Imaginations. One of these is the death process, which is represented by the three ravens. It is not only death that they prophesy however, but also its overcoming. Faithful John has overheard them and so is aware of the dangers threatening his king. And since the ravens also foretell that whoever reveals these dangers to the king will be turned to stone, Faithful John must keep his own counsel and ward off fate as best he can alone.

When upon his return the king jumps ashore, a chestnut horse comes galloping toward him. The young king is about to swing up onto the splendid steed when Faithful John suddenly intervenes by killing it with a lead bullet. Why? The ravens had foretold that if the king mounted the red horse, it would bear him away through the air. Then the young king would have vanished and never seen the princess again. It is this that Faithful John wishes to avert.

How is this episode to be interpreted in relation to the lead process? In Greek mythology the Imagination of liberated thought was represented by a winged horse—Pegasus. The depiction of this winged horse as chestnut-red can be interpreted as an enhanced Pegasus, though in a negative sense. It is an image of "flight of ideas"—mental distraction. But why does the tale incorporate this image?

The forces of Saturn make possible a body-free formation of thoughts, mental pictures, and memories.[10] Our thoughts are set free, given wings so to speak. When this process is given "free rein" and allowed to run wild, the human being can no longer formulate his thoughts with clarity and order. They "run away with him" and he suffers from absentmindedness, poor concentration and forgetfulness. Such a person will be in the middle of telling something, interrupt himself and begin to talk of something completely different. He is no longer able to listen, so conversation with him becomes

---

10   Steiner, *The Healing Process*, Nov. 16, 1923, The Hague.

impossible. This disease picture is seen in certain pathologies, as when arteriosclerosis affects the upper organization. The patient's reactions to incipient arteriosclerosis—generally inflammatory in nature—are well captured in the image of the red horse, for in all traditions the horse is used as an image for the forces of intelligence, and the winged horse for the power of thinking.

The imagery of this story can also be interpreted from another perspective. After the individuality has united with the Saturn forces, it progresses to the Jupiter sphere. The Jupiter sphere, along with the now assimilated forces of Saturn, gives form to the head forces of man. But when the Saturn forces act too strongly at this stage, the disposition is set for arteriosclerotic ailments. And when the disease process becomes manifest, lead is the remedy called for (*Plumbum mellitum D12,* for example), just as in the story the runaway Saturn process is overcome when Faithful John kills the horse by shooting it with a lead bullet.

The Lead Process and Self-destruction

Once the danger of the overly powerful Saturn process in the Jupiter sphere has been averted successfully, the individuality can enter the next planetary sphere, that of Mars. The story now shows how an excessive Saturn process acts in the Mars sphere, and at the same time how the Saturn process itself can prevent this deviation. As foretold by the ravens, when the young king enters the castle with his bride he spies the bridal robe lying on a salver in the great hall, appearing exactly as if it were woven of gold and silver. He is just about to pick it up when Faithful John shoves him aside, grasps it with gloves, and quickly carries it to the fire to burn it. For as he knows from the ravens' warning, the bridal robe only looks like silver and gold but in reality is nothing other than sulfur and pitch. If the prince were to put it on he would be burnt to the marrow of his bones.

When acting primarily on the organic level in conjunction with the Mars forces, the Saturn process causes breakdown and self-destruction in the lower (metabolic) pole. It is as though the organism were being burnt "to the marrow of its bones." This lead process in conjunction with the Mars forces is destructive heat; it is "pitch and sulfur." While the lead process in the nerve-sense system has the deadening effect that makes possible body-free sense perception and thinking, in the metabolic-limb system it causes breakdown, self-destruction, and hardening.[11]

This picture captures the side of the aging process that is associated with auto-aggressive, degenerative inflammatory processes—the loss of immune tolerance—in arteriosclerotic vascular alterations.[12] Certain allergic diseases caused by disorders in the realm of the life forces also belong here. From the perspective of anthroposophic medicine we are dealing here with an exactly defined imbalance in the integrating forces of the ether body—between the light and warmth ethers, on the one hand, and the life and tone ethers on the other. Therapeutically, lead in high potency is indicated for such diseases; the inner warmth of this metal plays an important role here as a kind of simile to the inflammatory processes. In the remedy *Plumbum mellitum* this aspect is strengthened by a second component—specially processed honey.

Most important in such disease forms, however, are the human forces of self-healing, which are expressed as spiritual warmth in the capacity for enthusiasm. Essentially, the aggressive, self-destructive lead forces can only be sublimated by the development of interests of the mind and spirit that permeate the organism with warmth and light. The seed of these healing forces should be planted and nurtured in childhood—for example, through an education filled with soul warmth. These seeds can then germinate and grow into spiritual fire, into enthusiasm for ideas and ideals, which counteract arteriosclerosis and related pathologies. The fairy tale expresses this cleansing force in the image of the fire within Faithful John can destroy the

11 Steiner, *From Elephants to Einstein...*, Jan. 19, 1924, Dornach.

12 Steiner, *An Occult Physiology*, Mar. 22, 1911, Prague.

pitch and sulfur forces. It is a true mercy that the lead process also has this aspect of warmth.

The Lead Process and Isolation

After passing through the Mars sphere, the individuality enters the sphere of the Sun, and if at this point it is dominated by the Saturn aspect (i.e., the influence of the lead process), then it is in mortal danger. It falls into darkening and isolation, particularly in the soul-spiritual realm; Saturn's darkness overshadows the light of the Sun sphere. At this moment the individuality experiences total isolation and sees itself separated out of the general order. Rudolf Steiner provides the following background:

> When anything at all—be it a solar system or man's circulatory system—is separated from the entire surrounding world and follows its own principle, it means that such a system violates and breaks the all-embracing outer laws, that it becomes independent of the outer laws and creates its own inner laws and its own rhythm.... This contradiction, which is simply a fact now, cannot be evened out until the rhythm that was established on the inside has completely adapted to the outer rhythm again.[13]

In other words, everything that takes on independence through the action of Saturn is immediately condemned by this action of Saturn to destroy itself. The fitting mythological image here is that of Saturn— or *Kronos*—consuming his own children.

The story depicts what we have just described as follows: the wedding celebration of the king and the Princess of the Golden Dwelling is underway. The dance begins. In the middle of the dance, the princess turns pale and falls to the ground as if dead. Faithful John, having learned from the ravens what to expect, springs in, lifts the princess, and bears her to her chamber. There he puts her on a bed, kneels down and sucks three drops of blood from her right breast and then spits it out. After this the princess recovers quickly.

---

13 P. Schleicher, J. Jahn and S. v. Sommoggy, "Immunologie und Arteriosklerose," *Schweizer Zeitschrift Ganzheitsmedizin* 4,1989.

What is intended by this episode? To understand the dance, we may say that the Saturn process is uniting with the Sun sphere, thus darkening it. Here the Saturn process manifests its sealing, delimiting, isolating qualities. This brings the individuality into danger of falling out of the universal order. Blood circulation is the human solar system, so to speak. The heart as the center of the organism is the mirror image of the Sun, and the circulation is the image of its sphere. Through the lead process the blood circulation is poisoned—and in fact, the story shows us the princess's circulatory system becoming gravely ill. Turning pale and fainting are signs that her circulation is in a bad way. The blood retreats. From her right breast the servant must suck three drops of blood, because in the right side of the body the venous element predominates—that is, the forces in the blood circulation that contain the process of fading and dying. When the poison is sucked out of the venous component of the circulation, the deadly poisoning process is overcome.

The Lead Process as a Death Process

Now that the danger of isolation in the Sun sphere has been averted, the wedding proper can take place. However, the lead process itself—Faithful John—has come to an end. This is represented in the story by John's death. Condemned to death as a traitor, he is given the opportunity to reveal his innocence to the king and explain the reasons for his actions. But since in doing so he must reveal the ravens' secrets, he instantly turns to stone as they had foretold.

The Lead Process as a Force of Resurrection

The royal couple mourns the undeserved death of their faithful servant. The king has the stone figure set up by his bed and weeps every time he sees it. This goes on for quite some time, until one day the stone begins to speak and informs the king how he can bring his servant to life again. He must kill his twin sons and smear the stone figure with their blood. Though he is initially terribly shocked at this thought, the king recognizes that he owes it to his faithful servant and does the deed. No sooner has stone-John been smeared with the blood than he comes back to life completely restored. And this first miracle is followed by a second: the resurrected servant in turn brings the dead children to life by smearing their wounds with their own blood. Here the fairy tale might end, but to reveal the lead process fully, the mother, too, is put to the test. Keeping his children and John hidden, the king explains to his wife why he had to kill them. Moreover, it proves that she, too, has fully incorporated the lead process, for in spite of her pain she does not reproach her husband and is able to affirm this sacrifice. Now the king can bring out the children and Faithful John, and all of them live happily ever after. Thus the tale ends.

These final images of the tale give a wonderfully vivid portrayal of the central motifs of the lead process as reflected in the human being. As we have noted, lead causes breakdown and hardening in the human being, a process that ultimately leads to mineralization of the bone. For this reason, lead preparations are employed therapeutically in cases of disturbed mineralization, as in rickets or bone metastases. In the skeletal system the lead process enters completely into spatial form; it "dies" into space and hardens into "stone." This, however, is not the end of the process; this is where it turns around and reawakens in the bone marrow as the regenerative forces of blood formation. Out of the center of the death process, where the living organism is given over wholly to mineralization, come re-enlivening and rejuvenation. Here new young blood cells are continually formed. This process, which is partially attributable to the lead process, is visible in the tale's powerful images for the soul: Faithful John's turning to stone and coming to life again rejuvenated by the children's blood.

The Lead Process and the Capacity for Enthusiasm

We may say that the height and quintessence of this fairy tale is sacrifice performed out of loyalty on the part of all concerned. All are capable of sacrifice: the faithful servant, the royal father and sublime mother; a mother who sacrifices her children sacrifices herself. Surely no human being can offer greater proof of self-sacrifice.

If one looks realistically at these scenes, what is asked of the king and queen is truly monstrous. For the king to rejoice at receiving the queen's approval of their children's sacrifice means essentially that self-sacrifice and unconditional loyalty are being raised to a principle. The loyalty of the servant can still be taken as fulfillment of duty, even if it goes far beyond the expected norm; but the queen's willingness to sacrifice her children cannot be expected out of any sense of duty, nor can it be understood out of feelings of pity, regret, or gratitude alone. This willingness comes from a deeper level that cannot be grasped by the mind, only in the deed. Thus the fairy tale plainly shows that feelings like gratitude and sadness are not enough, but that truly willed devotion is needed—even if one's own personal existence and future, here represented by the children, are blotted out. This is not the general principle of nature formulated by Goethe: "Life is her (Nature's) most exquisite invention and death her contrivance to get plenty of life." This is rather the principle of higher human development in the Christian sense—the principle of renewal through self-overcoming and even self-sacrifice.

To use Goethe's words again: "And until you've learned this truth, Die and Become!, you are but a dreary guest on a darkened Earth." When we study the scenes of the tale in this manner, we become acquainted with yet another aspect of the Saturn process that is connected with the spleen. In the previous section we spoke of the lead process as the power of resurrection, which takes place through hematopoiesis. Now we come to the process in which the blood (actually the red corpuscles) is broken down or "dies" once more in the spleen. At the same time, this decay and death process in the spleen is also associated with spreading a certain "spiritual warmth," a tendency toward spiritualization and enthusiasm.

Thus the spleen is the organ that provides the physical basis for enthusiasm, enabling the human being to develop a fire for ideals.

This fire not only takes hold of our conscious mind, our thought world, but characteristically also draws us into action even at the cost of the greatest personal sacrifices. In other words, with this phase the lead process draws us fully into the future; and so we can say that the Saturn process, though rooted in past-orientation, also reveals important future aspects: it allows human beings to recognize ideals whose realization requires complete disregard for one's own person. In this way human action is not only bound up with the past but just as firmly pointed toward the future.

Soul Dispositions in Connection with the Lead Process

In "Faithful John," we recognize imaginatively not only motifs of the lead dynamic, but also find a soul study of the personality type influenced by the Saturn sphere. We will focus on this aspect later, but let us merely point briefly to the soul traits we encounter in therapeutic experience, as well as in the imaginations of our fairy tale. These are the very soul qualities found in the essential being of the Saturn sphere, which Steiner describes as past-oriented, inward, and profundity. Those in whom they appear internalize the past so that it determines their behavior from the very depths of their souls.

This gives such disposed individuals an earnest tenor of soul that is far from superficiality, seeking the meaning in everything. The behavior of Saturn types is therefore marked by a sense of duty and perseverance. Their relationship to the spiritual world is inward and alive. It is the great ideals such as freedom, justice, and loyalty that fan the fire of enthusiasm in the souls of such people. When personal renunciation or sacrifice is required to realize these ideals, they show no hesitation. Their seriousness, formed by past experiences, contains at the same time a future orientation; they believe in a future in which they can see their ideals realized. Thus their past-oriented nature clearly contains germinal future aspects within itself. In the figure of Faithful John we can recognize an exact character description of the Saturn type.

The Fairy Tale and Lead as a Remedy

The tale of "Faithful John" has given us a picture of the entire lead process—both its normal and its pathological action in the human being. The lead process, and with it the remedy *Plumbum,* is illustrated for us in vivid fairy-tale images. Through its depth and spirituality this fairy tale can be an unending source of knowledge. In the chapter on character typology we will return to this story and draw further insights from it. One interpretation of a fairy tale never exhausts the living source; fresh insights are always to be gained.

Whether an interpretation of a fairy tale is true or false is not a question that can be easily answered. In fact, it may not be a useful question at all. The critical question is whether an interpretation proves fruitful and means something to the reader or listener. In our comparison of the lead process and the tale of Faithful John one or another aspect of the interpretation may appear questionable, but this is not critical regarding the conclusions we have reached. What matters is if through it, the reader has gained a vivid picture of and an inner connection to the lead process. If the interpretation has been fruitful in this sense, then it has its justification.

It should go without saying that in the process of interpreting this fairy tale medically, one must hold to the established therapeutic experiences with lead remedies. The insights gained must be coherent and must prove valid when applied in practice; for this to hold true the interpretations can never be arbitrary or speculative. What we have established here in this first fairy-tale-based remedy description will hold true for those to follow.

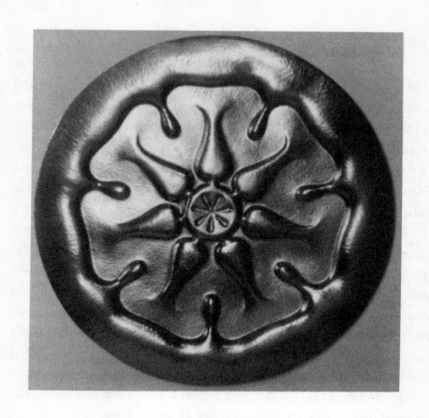

Sun Seal

Tin as a Remedy: "The Goose Girl"

There once lived an old queen whose husband had been dead for many years, and she had a beautiful daughter. When the princess grew up she was promised in marriage to a prince who lived far away. When the time came for her to be married, and she had to depart for the distant kingdom, the old queen packed up for her many costly vessels and utensils of silver and gold, and trinkets also of gold and silver, and cups and jewels—in short, everything that belonged to a royal dowry, for she loved her child with all her heart.

She likewise assigned to her a chambermaid, who was to ride with her and deliver her into the hands of the bridegroom. Each received a horse for the journey. The princess's horse, called Falada, was able to speak. When the hour of departure came, the old mother went into her bedroom, took a small knife, and cut her fingers with it until they bled. Then she held out a small white cloth and let three drops of blood fall into it. She gave them to her daughter, saying, "Take good care of these. They will be of service to you on your way."

Thus they sorrowfully took leave of each other. The princess put the cloth into her bosom, mounted her horse, and set off for her bridegroom. After they had ridden for a while, she felt a burning thirst and said to her chambermaid, "Dismount, and take my cup that you brought with you for me and get me some water from the brook, for I would like a drink."

"If you are thirsty," said the chambermaid, "get off your horse yourself and lie down near the water and drink. I won't be your servant."

So in her great thirst the princess dismounted, bent down over the water in the brook and drank; and she was not allowed to drink from the golden cup. Then she said, "Oh, Lord," and the three drops of blood answered, "If your mother knew this, her heart would break in two."

But the king's daughter was humble. She said nothing and remounted her horse. They rode some miles farther. The day was warm, the sun beat down, and she grew thirsty again. When they came to a stream of water, she again called to her chambermaid, "Dismount and give me some water in my golden cup," for she had long ago forgotten the girl's evil words.

But the chambermaid said still more haughtily, "If you want a drink, get it yourself. I won't be your servant."

Then in her great thirst the king's daughter dismounted, bent over the flowing water, wept, and said, "Oh, Lord," and the drops of blood again replied, "If your mother knew this, her heart would break in two."

As she was thus drinking, leaning over the stream, the cloth with the three drops of blood fell from her bosom and floated away with the water without her noticing, so great were her concerns. However, the chambermaid saw what happened, and she rejoiced to think that she now had power over the bride, for by losing the drops of blood the princess had become weak and powerless.

When she wanted to mount her horse again, the one called Falada, the chambermaid said, "I belong on Falada. You belong on my nag," and the princess had to accept it.

Then, with many harsh words, the chambermaid ordered the princess to take off her royal clothing and put on the chambermaid's shabby clothes. In the end, the princess had to swear under the open heaven that she would not say one word of this to anyone at the royal court. If she had not taken this oath, she would have been killed on the spot. Falada saw everything and remembered it well.

The chambermaid now climbed onto Falada, and the true bride onto the bad horse, and thus they traveled on until they finally arrived at the royal palace. There was great rejoicing over their arrival, and the prince ran ahead to meet them and, thinking she was his bride, lifted the chambermaid from her horse.

She was led upstairs while the real princess was left standing below. Then the old king looked out of the window, saw her waiting in the courtyard, and noticed how fine and delicate and beautiful she was. At once he went to the royal apartment and asked the bride about the girl she had with her who was standing down below in the courtyard and who she was.

"I picked her up on my way for a companion. Give the girl some work to do, so she won't stand about idly."

However, the old king had no work for her and knew of nothing else to say but, "I have a little boy who tends the geese. She can help him." The boy was called Little Conrad, and the true bride had to help him tend geese.

Soon after, the false bride said to the young king, "Dearest husband, I beg you to do me a favor."

He answered, "I will do so gladly."

"Then send for the butcher of useless animas and have the head cut off the horse I rode on, for it angered me on the way." In truth, she was afraid that the horse might tell how she had behaved toward the king's daughter.

Thus it happened that faithful Falada had to die. The real princess heard about this, and she secretly promised to pay the butcher a piece of gold if he would perform a small service for her. In the town was a large dark gateway through which she had to pass with the geese each morning and evening. Would he be so good as to nail Falada's head beneath the gateway, so that she might see him again and again?

The butcher's helper promised to do so. He cut off the head and nailed it securely beneath the dark gateway.

Early the next morning, as she and Conrad drove their flock out beneath this gateway, she said in passing, "Alas, Falada, hanging there!"

The head answered, "Alas, young queen passing by, if your mother knew this, her heart would break in two."

Then they went still further out of the town, driving their geese into the country. And when they came to the meadow, she sat and unbound her hair of pure gold. Conrad saw it, was delighted how it glistened, and wanted to pluck out a few hairs.

She said, "Blow, wind, blow. Take Conrad's hat, and make him chase it until I have braided my hair and tied it up again." Then such a strong wind came up that it blew Conrad's hat across the fields, and he had to run after it. When he returned, she was already finished combing and putting up her hair, so he could not get even one strand. Thus, Conrad became angry and would not speak to her, and they tended the geese until evening and they went home.

The next morning when they were driving the geese out through the dark gateway, the maiden said, "Alas, Falada, hanging there!"

Falada answered, "Alas, young queen passing by, if this your mother knew, her heart would break in two." She sat down again in the field and began combing out her hair.

When Conrad ran up and tried to take hold of some, she quickly said, "Blow, wind, blow. Take Conrad's hat and make him chase it until I have braided my hair and tied it up again."

Again the wind blew, taking the hat off his head and far away. Conrad had to run after it, and when he came back she had already put up her hair, and he could not get a single strand. Then they tended the geese until evening.

That evening, after they had returned home, Conrad went to the old king and said, "I won't tend geese with that girl any longer."

"Why not?" asked the old king.

"Because she angers me all day long."

The old king ordered him to tell what it was that she did to him. Conrad said, "In the morning when we pass beneath the dark gateway with the flock, there is a horse's head on the wall, and she says to it, 'Alas, Falada, hanging there!' And the head replies, 'Alas, young queen passing by, if this your mother knew, her heart would break in two." Then Conrad went on to tell what happened at the goose pasture, and how he had to chase his hat.

The old king ordered him to drive his flock out again the next day. As soon as morning came, he himself sat behind the dark gateway and heard how the girl spoke to Falada's head. Then he followed her out into the country meadow and hid himself in a thicket. There, he soon saw with his own eyes the goose girl and the goose boy bringing their flock and how after a while she sat down and took down her hair, which glistened brightly.

She said, "Blow, wind, blow. Take Conrad's hat, and make him chase it until I have braided my hair and tied it up again." Then came a blast of wind and carried off Conrad's hat, so that he had to run far away, while the maiden went on quietly combing and braiding her hair, all of which the king observed. Then, quite unseen, he went away, and when the goose girl returned home in the evening, he called her aside and asked why she did all these things.

"I am not allowed to tell you, nor can I reveal my sorrows to any human being, for I have sworn under the open heavens not to do so. If I had not so sworn, I would have been killed."

He urged her and left her no peace, but he could get nothing from her. Finally he said, "If you will not tell me anything, then tell your sorrows to the iron stove there," and he went away.

So she crept into the iron stove and began to cry sorrowfully, pouring out her whole heart. She said, "Here I sit, abandoned by the whole world, although I am the daughter of a king. A false chambermaid forced me to take off my royal clothes, and she has taken my place with my bridegroom. Now I have to do common work as a goose girl. If my mother knew this, her heart would break in two."

The old king was standing outside listening by the stovepipe, and he heard what she said. Then he came back inside and asked her to come out of the stove. Then they dressed her in royal clothes, and it was marvelous how beautiful she was.

39

The old king summoned his son and revealed to him that he had a false bride who was only a chambermaid, but that the true one was standing there, the one who had been a goose girl. The young king rejoiced with all his heart when he saw her beauty and virtue. A great feast was made ready, to which all the people and all good friends were invited.

At the head of the table sat the bridegroom with the king's daughter on one side of him and the chambermaid on the other. However, the chambermaid was deceived, for she did not recognize the princess in her dazzling attire. After they had eaten and drank and were in a good mood, the old king asked the chambermaid, as a riddle, what punishment a person deserved who had deceived her master in such and such a way, then told the whole story, asking finally, "What sentence does such a person deserve?"

The false bride said, "She deserves no better fate than to be stripped stark naked and put in a barrel studded inside with sharp nails. Two white horses should be hitched to it and they should drag her along through one street after another until she is dead."

"You are the one," said the old king, "and you have pronounced your own sentence. Thus shall it be done to you."

After the sentence had been carried out, the young king married his true bride, and they ruled over their kingdom in peace and happiness.[1]

~

After passing through the Saturn sphere on its path to incarnation, the "I" enters the Jupiter sphere, which is associated with the metal tin. We will now explore the tin process and its therapeutic uses based on "The Goose Girl"; but for a better understanding of the imaginative pictures of this tale we must first examine how the tin process acts in the human being.

---

1   Trans. by Margaret Hunt (1884), revised and corrected by D. L. Ashliman http://www.pitt.edu/~dash/ashliman.html; emended by the translator.

The Tin Process in the Human Being

The tin or Jupiter process is the great sculptor in the human—and the animal—organism. Bernard Lievegoed writes, "If the sublime forms of the skeleton are created by Saturn as a naked image of the spirit, then the soft forms of fluid beauty surrounding this skeleton are Jupiter's handiwork. If Jupiter alone were at work in us, by the age of fourteen we would all be the most beautiful Greek sculptures, every pose and gesture breathing pure soul. We would be images of Apollo or Venus, for Jupiter's plastic power bears a sublime ordering wisdom. This wisdom is manifest in the marvelous structure of our organs, which it sculpts out of the watery element."[1]

It is the cosmic principles at work in Jupiter's forming and modeling that give rise to the curves and arches in our organism. Through the Jupiter process, the arc of the heavens finds its reflection in the rounded forms of our organs. Our domed forehead and the smooth, round balls of our joints reveal this principle at work. Internally, the relation between solid and fluid is Jupiter's sphere of action. Thus, the tin process regulates the relation between fluid and solid in the formation of the brain and cerebrospinal fluid in childhood.[2] When this Jupiter dynamic is not properly controlled, the result is either hydrocephaly (fluid dominating) or a hardening that leads to premature aging (solid dominating). The joints with their synovial fluid and cartilage are another particular sphere of its activity. If the fluid phase is dominant here, it results in loose, swollen joints that sprain easily; if the hardening tendency is dominant, degenerative diseases of the joints are likely to develop.

There is one organ that wonderfully expresses the wisdom-filled cosmic principles of the tin process, though less in its formation than in its chemistry and fine metabolism: the liver.[3] The wisdom

---

1   Lievegoed, *Man on the Threshold.*

2   Steiner, *Introducing Anthroposophical Medicine,* Mar. 27, 1920, Dornach.

3   Steiner, *An Occult Physiology,* Mar. 28, 1911, Prague.

41

that permeates the activity of our brains and enables us to grasp the lawfulness of natural phenomena is also at work (quite unconsciously to us) in the metabolic etheric realm of the liver. Thus on the one hand, the Jupiter process ensures that all the subtle-material processes in the liver proceed in an orderly way and do not flow into one another, while on the other it enables us to gain a true mental grasp of the ordering principles and overarching connections in the world. This faculty of the grand overview belongs to the Jupiter dynamic. It allows for the meaningful ordering of things, so that the most disparate processes can take place alongside one another without causing chaos.

Following high cosmic laws, Jupiter acts symmetrically. It is the Jupiter forces that give rise to the organizational principle of left and right. The precondition for the operation of this principle is a balanced relation between fluid and solid, and in regulating this balance the liver is a critical organ. For example it also regulates thirst, a fact that becomes significant in understanding certain points in the fairy tale.

The Tin Process and the Primary Motifs of the Tale

If "Faithful John" can be said to have a single primary motif—loyalty—then it will be necessary to speak of two primary motifs in "The Goose Girl"—a pair of polar traits represented by two different characters, the princess and the chambermaid. It should be understood that as fairy-tale figures these two do not stand for rivals in an external sense, but for divergent inner-human forces that manifest both in the soul and in the bodily realm. The princess and the chambermaid embody a dynamic that is operative in every human being—two sides of ourselves. Let us examine it.

The princess's dejection and weakness, her lack of self-confidence and self-assertiveness, all point to a weak tin process, while the chambermaid's domineering, presumptuous, ostentatious character speaks clearly of one that is excessively strong. It lies in the character of the tin process always to move between extremes; yet only the balancing of these contrasts brings harmony to both the soul and bodily realms. A healthy tin process can be found only in between—in a balance between the soul attitudes of the princess and the chambermaid.

In the lead process, all was oriented to the past. A healthy tin process, in contrast, is directed toward the present—toward what lies between past and future.[4] In this tale the past figures in the royal lineage and the caring devotion of the princess's mother, who gives her daughter a cloth with three drops of her own blood to take on her journey. The future beckons from afar in the planned wedding, the aim of the journey that will take the princess and chambermaid to the bridegroom. On the way, however, the princess loses the power drawn from heredity—her past—when she loses the drops of blood. And her future is contested by the chambermaid who usurps her role and claims the bridegroom for herself. How is this to be interpreted?

When the tin process is ineffective, the soul remains bound to the past; when too strong, it is completely focused on the future. What it must learn is to live consciously in the present. A healthy tin process forms the foundation for effectiveness in the moment. This is pictorially illustrated toward the end of the story, when the princess crawls into the iron stove, indicating that she has united with the forces of iron and is beginning to assert herself in the here-and-now. Self-assertion in the present is thus a characteristic made possible for human beings by proper action of the Jupiter sphere.

To penetrate the specifically physiological aspects of the tin process we must enter wholly into the imaginative language of the fairy tale. In harmony with cosmic laws the Jupiter dynamic forms the head; and the formation of the front of the head specifically offers us a faculty of thought that embodies wisdom. This aspect, as we shall see later, is presented in the speaking horse Falada. After forming the head, the tin process sinks into the organism and assumes its seat

---

4   Steiner, *Initiationswissenschaft und Sternenerkenntnis*, July 27, 1923, Dornach.

of activity in the liver. Here its formative power is transformed into a wisdom-filled functional guidance of chemical metabolic processes. Only now can the liver produce the energy that gives the muscles the power of movement, thus enabling the organism to exert physical power. The fairy tale has chosen fitting images to represent this: the princess tending geese and commanding the wind to blow off the hat of her meddlesome companion Conrad, forcing him to chase after it. Once the tin process has engaged in the liver metabolism, it enters into connection with the iron processes at work there, which produces a further strengthening. In the language of the fairy tale, the princess finds the courage to recognize and face the demands of the moment. Only now is she able to expose the false chamber-maid—that is, manage the present in such a way that the future, her bridegroom, would belong to her. Later we will find additional support for this interpretation of the plot.

This preliminary overview of the significant motifs of the tale has highlighted characteristic aspects of the tin process in the organism. A clear correspondence between them is already evident, but as we investigate the specific images more closely below, we will need to gain an even fuller understanding of the tin process if we are to perceive it clearly in the imaginations of the fairy tale.

Cosmic Principles of the Tin Process

The opening of the story speaks of a princess who has only a mother, her father having died long ago. The mother in particular is mentioned again and again in the course of the story. Altogether, we are struck by the emphasis placed on the feminine element in this tale. So if we are told at the start of the tale that the princess has a special connection to her mother, we may say that the princess represents particularly those forces that are aligned with the maternal line of heredity. Now, it is the cosmic element that is chiefly manifested in the female stream of heredity, the earthly in the male. Thus the limb organization owes more to the paternal side, the head organization

44

more to the maternal side, since the rounding cosmic form forces of the tin process act through it.[5] Moreover, by repeatedly referring to the maternal element, the tale expresses this interrelationship: tin process / maternal stream of heredity / cosmic formative forces.

The tin process makes it possible for the cosmic forces of structure and order to be guided into the earthly. Mediating between the fluid element of cosmic wisdom and the solid element of earth, it establishes a balance between them. When this process is disturbed, the organism either remains too attached to the watery element or becomes hardened and rigid. The character picture of the princess points to the former—to a tin process clinging to the cosmic. The latter—excessive hardening—is embodied by the chambermaid. Thus in a sense the princess and the chambermaid represent the relation between left and right, with the princess standing for the left and the chambermaid for the right side of our being. The right, in this picture, is the earthly, the strong, the domineering or even arrogant side; the left is the cosmic, the emotional, the sensitive and by tendency the weak side.

Now, what is the horse's role? The horse is the creature that came into being when man was first endowed with the forces of thought[6]— an event which itself was made possible by the tin process. It is this process that is imaginatively portrayed in the story by the speaking horse named Falada, and it plays quite a significant role; Falada is a representation of human intelligence and power of thought. How is this to be understood? According to Rudolf Steiner's investigations, the horse came into being at the time in Earth's development when human beings were gifted with the power of thought—that is, when human intelligence took form. This happened in the middle of what Spiritual Science calls the Atlantean period. As a new human body develops, the tin process forms the front of the head containing the cerebrum, thus making possible human intelligence and thinking.

---

5   Steiner, *Education for Special Needs*, July 3, 1924, Dornach.

6   Steiner, *The Christian Mystery*, Oct. 13, 1906, Leipzig.

This significant aspect of the tin process is aptly represented in the image of a speaking horse. If the Saturn sphere is the memory in the planetary system, then the Jupiter sphere can be described as the realm of the thought faculty. Here the "I" receives the germinal capacity that develops into the power of discriminating thought in Earth existence.

The Polarity of the Tin Process

On the journey to her bridegroom, the princess is seized by thirst. In other words, her organism yearns to keep dwelling in the fluid phase, to retain its original relationship to the cosmic forces and not dry up. Her fluid-organism makes its presence felt, thus pointing to a disturbed tin process. A symptom in the remedy picture of tin is thirst, and thirst is connected with the liver metabolism.[7]

With the appearance of thirst, the polar relationship of the princess and her chambermaid becomes more obvious; their first conflict arises. The chambermaid will not draw water for the princess. She does not want to be her maid at all, but to assume the princess's role herself. The over-strong and the over-weak weak tin processes collide. As noted above, when the tin process leads too deeply into hardening, this is when the traits of arrogance, imperiousness, presumption, pomposity, and ostentation appear. When on the other hand the tin process clings to the cosmic, the consequence is generalized weakness and particularly lack of self-assertiveness. The polarization becomes still more obvious when the princess feels thirst for the second time. Again the chambermaid refuses to draw water from the stream. As the princess does it herself, she loses the cloth with the three drops of blood that her mother had given her. The chambermaid does not fail to notice this and perceives that she now has power over the princess. She forces her to turn over her royal garments and even her horse Falada. How does this episode relate to the tin process?

---

7   Steiner, "Notizen zum ersten Ärztekurs," in *Beiträge zur Rudolf Steiner Gesamtausgabe*, #35, Michaelmas 1971, Dornach.

With the loss of her mother's blood drops (i.e., loss of maternal forces), the princess's complete weakness becomes fully evident. Let us approach this from the point of view of child development. After birth the child is still largely protected by its mother's milk. If the mother is healthy, her milk gives the child strength and protection from outer influences. Mother's milk can be called the cosmic nourishment of the child. The moment this form of nourishment is withdrawn, the child is totally subject to the stream of earthly food. Now earthly hardening can gain the upper hand over cosmic plasticity. The earthly tin process seizes power and gains control over the developing human being, while the cosmic principle succumbs to these forces. In this sense, the three blood drops correspond to mother's milk. They are her provision for the way, as mother's milk is the provision for our "earthly journey." The moment the protection of the maternal forces ceases, the child must develop its own defenses to survive. It must confront earthly circumstances and influences. This is shown pictorially to us in the conflict between the princess and the chambermaid. Initially the earthly principle gains the upper hand; the chambermaid is able to appropriate the role of princess.

The Double

Their roles now reversed, the pair continues their journey to the bridegroom's court. The chambermaid has become the princess's double, so to speak, and now has power over her. In this way they arrive at the bridegroom's castle, the princess as chambermaid and the chambermaid as seeming princess. The young king fails to see through the role reversal and believes the seeming princess to be his bride. Only the old king, who might be interpreted as the higher Self, is not deceived and has a sense that there is something special about this "chambermaid." Unlike the young king he does not allow himself to be impressed by outer appearances. The ordinary self takes appearance for reality, but the higher Self intuitively recognizes the cosmic background. It can sense a spiritual kinship with the cosmic and cannot be blinded by the external show of the double. The ordinary self quickly becomes entangled in the earthly world—so much that it easily takes this side for the essential reality.

The Liver

The true princess must now tend the geese, and at the bidding of the false bride Falada is killed. The princess manages to arrange for Falada's head to be hung under the arch of the gateway. When the self identifies with the earthly, the earthly gains influence on its thought processes. Wisdom-filled thinking must die away, as we see depicted in the killing of Falada. The king (the young "I") is appointed by the (false) princess to arrange the killing of Falada. In other words, the self lets the forces of wisdom represented by Falada die in its thinking. The cosmic tin process, however, saves the head, which lives on under the dark archway. Each morning it enters into dialog with the princess as she walks out to the field to tend the geese. In other words, the princess must leave the domain of the court. The court, where the false bride now reigns and controls the young king, can be interpreted as the head, which the cosmic tin process must leave. The cosmic tin process sinks into the body, taking "Falada" along as far as the archway, which is the limit of the sway of the court—i.e., of thinking. Wisdom-filled thinking has been displaced to the threshold between consciousness and unconsciousness, an area where it is dark.

In the image of the princess tending the geese outside the gates we recognize the tin process engaging in the liver and acting in its chemistry. The goose can be recognized as a symbol for the liver processes. Metabolically, the entire animal is oriented toward the liver process, which gives it its particular chemical subtlety. (It is no accident that geese produce the finest liver *pâté*.) The image of the Goose Girl combing and braiding her golden hair in the field also has a connection to the liver functions; it is an image of the tin process as it penetrates the activity of the liver and orders the metabolic processes there with its wisdom. (In "Iron Hans" we will recognize the golden hair as an imaginative picture of the etheric body, particularly as it acts in the liver.)

As the tin process moves down from the head pole to the metabolic pole, the focus of tin activity switches from external forming to the internal chemistry. The wisdom-borne tin activity vanishes from the outward beauty and order and reappears in the inner chemical activity of the liver. The pure formative principle of the tin process in the head would lead to formal perfection, but at the same time to rigidity and inner weakness. This shifting of the tin process into chemical activity opens the way to overcoming rigidity and weakness; it is the liver's chemical activity that supplies us with the energy for movement. The muscle draws substances from the liver that enable it to contract and expand. Physical weakness is overcome and strength flows into the body's movement. In the fairy tale, the element of movement is expressed in the Goose Girl's appeal to the wind, which blows away Conrad's hat. Conrad must jump up and run after it—in other words, he must "really get moving."

The Tin Process and the Power of Iron

From Conrad, the old king learns what has been happening under the dark archway and out on the field. He asks the princess the meaning of these goings-on, but she says nothing; she will reveal her secret only in the iron stove. The "fire" of the iron process brings out her true nature. Iron allows the universal to unite with the individual. The tin process is this wisdom-filled universal and can be individualized by the fiery iron forces. Alone, the tin process lacks individualizing power on the earthly plane. This is supplied when it unites with the iron process; now the cosmic tin process gains the power of self-assertion.

This power exposes the double. The false bride is recognized for the arrogant pretender that she is. The "I" (the old king) informs the self (the young king) which one is the true royal bride. Thus the iron process is the undoing of the false bride. She is put into a barrel lined with sharp iron nails and rolled to death. The barrel is drawn by two white horses. Like every detail of a fairy tale, this image must be seen in the context of the whole and interpreted as a corresponding motif. We may interpret the white horses as purified reason and purified thinking. Purified thinking is able to recognized the double in its workings and thus deprive it of its life.

Disease Pictures and "The Goose Girl"

Let us now consider the tale from a medical perspective—that is, in terms of its relation to *Stannum* as a remedy. It may at first seem surprising that the Jupiter process is not embodied by a male character. The name of Jupiter (or Zeus) evokes images of the Greek god of that name or of majestic fatherly divinities. Great men such as Goethe are also often associated with wisdom-filled thinking. In fact, however, these figures do not embody the Jupiter process alone, but the other planetary processes as well. Thus, the god Jupiter/Zeus also displays characteristics of the Mercury process. Among the Greek gods it is Pallas Athena, goddess of wisdom, art and knowledge, who embodies the pure Jupiter process. And she was born out of the forehead of Zeus.

The homeopathic remedy picture of *Stannum* also displays a specific relationship to the female sex, but no obvious one to the male. Thus, certain illnesses of the female reproductive organs can be cured with *Stannum* in potentized form. Here are two typical examples of cases where *Stannum* preparations are helpful.[8] A woman who once suffered from severe neuralgia reports that since these pains ceased she has had abundant, thick, yellow or green discharge. Another patient reports that her monthly periods tend to come too early and profusely and that she has a sensation of uterine prolapse.

That tin has a stronger essential connection to woman than to man is symbolized in the tale simply by the fact that the two main

---

8   Tylor Kent, *Arzneimittelbilder—Vorlesungen zur homöopathischen Materia Medica* (Drug images lectures on Homeopathic Materia Medica).

characters are both women. After all, it can be said as a general truth that the feminine represents the cosmic aspect of the human being; thus the Jupiter process, as a force of order and wisdom, has a closer connection to the female than to the male.

Depression and the Tin Process

In the character traits of the princess and the chambermaid we recognize two disease pictures for which *Stannum* is therapeutically indicated. The picture embodied by the princess is one of comprehensive weakness. Her weakness increases and finally reaches a point of total defenselessness when she loses the three drops of blood. She yields without struggle to the power-mongering of the chambermaid. It so happens that pronounced psychic weakness and low energy are also primary features of the remedy picture for *Stannum*.

The picture also includes physical exhaustion, generalized muscular weakness, and excessive thirst. As thirst is regulated by the liver, elevated thirst can be an indication of liver dysfunction. (Thirst itself is not a specific indication of a disturbed tin dynamic, as it appears in numerous other ailments.) In addition, hypochondriac traits are encountered in *Stannum* patients. When the princess repeatedly bewails her unhappy lot to Falada's head in the dark archway, one might say she is engaging in an ineffectual monologue with her own head forces that revolves solely around her own suffering. This is a pattern that can be classified medically as hypochondria; and hypochondria is another syndrome associated with an unbalanced liver metabolism. As to the image of Falada's head suspended beneath the archway, this can be connected with yet another important aspect of the *Stannum* remedy picture.

Strangely, although only his head is left, Falada seems to be still alive. The image is comparable to a condition in which a patient is able to feel only his head, losing awareness of the rest of his organism. This occurs in certain types of headaches—neuralgia of the head nerves. The headaches recur every morning and can be so intense that they lead to mental stupor. *Stannum* can be an effective remedy in such cases.

Mania and the Tin Process

Now let us turn to the chambermaid, the false bride. She displays a certain toughness of character that is directed purely to externals, to power. The traits we recognize in her—arrogance, imposture, domineering, and ostentation—all point to a heightened tin process. When these tendencies are exaggerated, they lead to what is known as "flight of ideas" and manic agitation. At that point we are clearly in the pathological realm, which is an apt way of describing the false bride's condition at the wedding. In her self-infatuation and distraction she no longer recognizes the princess sitting next to her, and when the old king recounts her own story to her in the form of a riddle, she is incapable of connecting it with herself and pronounces her own death sentence. For manic agitation *Stannum met.* D3-6 is indicated.

Left and Right: Two Sides of the Jupiter Process

To understand the contrasting poles represented by the princess and the chambermaid, we need to recall that the tin process forms the front of the head. The front of the head contains the cerebrum, which consists of two hemispheres, a right and a left. The two hemispheres have different functions and thus mediate a differentiated understanding of reality.[9] The right brain is geared more to holistic, spatial and intuitive perception, while the left brain facilitates the analytic, intellectual, and temporal faculties. The right brain is directed more toward the cosmic and mediates spiritual thinking, while the left brain is more related to the earthly and is connected with pragmatic, intellectual thinking. It appears that in women the right brain is more highly developed, and in men the left brain. The healthy tin process

---

9   John C. Eccles, "Hirn und Bewusstsein" [Brain and Consciousness], Mannheimer Forum 1977/78. *Ein Panomrama der Naturwissenchaften*, Studenreihe Boehringer Mannheim.

has to do with this apportionment of left and right, connecting and balancing the two sides. And this polarity, too, is visible in the two female characters of our fairy tale—the princess reflecting characteristics of the right brain and the chambermaid those of the left.

Yet not all disease pictures that call for *Stannum* are so clearly reflected in the fairy tale as those discussed so far. *Stannum* is also an important remedy for degenerative and deforming joint diseases such as *Arthrosis deformans*.[10] It is more difficult to find a connection to this in the tale. The element of movement is captured in the image of Conrad running after his hat all day long, but this alone is not sufficiently specific to be connected with degenerative joint disease. However, if we look at this disease picture not only as a locally defined phenomenon but in connection with gesture as a movement sequence, then we can make a certain link to the fairy tale. The *Stannum* process creates cosmic, rounded feminine forms of exalted beauty. That is the aspect that figures at the beginning of the tale in its emphasis on the royal feminine stream of heredity. On the other hand the *Stannum* process also guides subtle chemical activity, particularly in the liver. This combination of form-giving and chemical activity gives rise to formed movement—that is, to movement as gesture. As the movement apparatus ages, becoming insufficiently ensouled and falling into rigidity and mineralization, it can be re-enlivened by stimulating the *Stannum* process in the organism. And it is specifically the round joints that this addresses. Thus by taking account of the tale in its wholeness we can establish a connection to the joints as well.

---

10   I.e., osteoarthritis (TN).

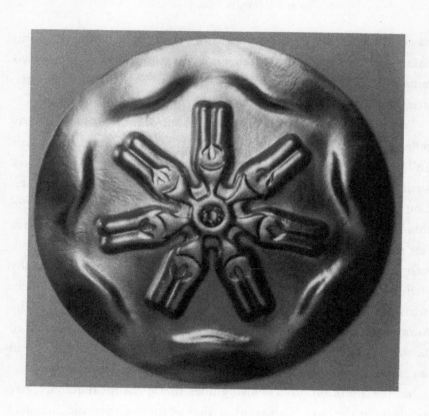

Moon Seal

IRON AS A REMEDY: "IRON HANS"

There was once upon a time a king who had a great forest near his palace, full of all kinds of wild animals. One day he sent out a hunter to shoot him a roe, but he did not come back. "Perhaps some accident has befallen him," said the king, and the next day he sent out two more hunters who were to search for him, but they too stayed away.

Then, on the third day, he sent for all his hunters and said, "Scour the whole forest through, and do not give up until you have found all three." But of these also, none came home again, none were seen again. From that time forth, no one would any longer venture into the forest, and it lay there in deep stillness and solitude, and nothing was seen of it, but sometimes an eagle or a hawk flying over it. This lasted for many years, when an unknown hunter announced himself to the king as seeking a situation, and offered to go into the dangerous forest. The king, however, would not give his consent and said, "It is not safe in there. I fear it would fare with you no better than with the others, and you would never come out again."

The hunter replied, "Lord, I will venture it at my own risk, of fear I know nothing." The hunter therefore went with his dog to the forest. It was not long before the dog fell in with some game on the way and wanted to pursue it; but hardly had the dog run two steps when it stood before a deep pool, could go no farther, and a naked arm stretched itself out of the water, seized it, and drew it under. When the hunter saw that, he went back and fetched three men to come with buckets and bail out the water. When they could see to the bottom there lay a wild man whose body was brown like rusty iron and whose hair hung over his face down to his knees. They bound him with cords

55

and led him away to the castle. There was great astonishment over the wild man; the king, however, had him put in an iron cage in his courtyard and forbade the door to be opened on pain of death, and the queen herself was to take the key into her keeping. And from this time forth everyone could again go into the forest with safety.

The king had a son of eight years, who was once playing in the courtyard. As he was playing, his golden ball fell into the cage. The boy ran thither and said, "Give me my ball."

"Not until you have opened the door for me," answered the man.

"No," said the boy, "I will not do that. The king has forbidden it," and ran away.

The next day he went again and asked for his ball. The wild man said, "Open my door," but the boy would not.

On the third day the king rode out hunting, and the boy went once more and said, "I cannot open the door even if I wished. I do not have the key."

Then the wild man said, "It lies under your mother's pillow; you can get it there."

The boy, who wanted his ball back cast all thought to the winds, and brought the key. The door opened with difficulty, and the boy pinched his fingers. Once it was open, the wild man stepped out, gave him the golden ball, and hurried away. The boy became afraid and called after him, "Oh, wild man, do not go away or I shall be beaten!"

The wild man turned back, took him up, set him on his shoulder, and stepped hastily into the forest.

When the king came home, he observed the empty cage and asked the queen how that happened. She knew nothing about it and sought the key, but it was gone. She called the boy, but no one answered. The king sent out people to seek him in the fields, but they did not find him. Then he could easily guess what had happened and much grief reigned in the royal court.

When the wild man had once more reached the dark forest, he took the boy down from his shoulder and said to him, "You will never see your father and mother again, but I will keep you with me, for you have set me free and I have compassion on you. If you do all I ask, you will fare well. I have enough treasure and gold—more than anyone in the world." He made a bed of moss for the boy, on which he slept, and the next morning the man took him to a well and said, "Behold, the gold well is as bright and clear as crystal. You shall sit beside it, and take care that nothing falls into it, or it will be polluted. I will come every evening to see if you have obeyed my order."

The boy placed himself by the edge of the well and often saw a golden fish or a golden snake show itself in it and took care that nothing fell in. As he sat, his finger hurt him so violently that he involuntarily put it into the water. He drew it quickly out again, but saw that it was quite gilded, and whatsoever pains he took to wash the gold off all was useless.

In the evening Iron Hans returned, looked at the boy, and said, "What has happened to the well?"

"Nothing, nothing," he answered, and held his finger behind his back so that the man would not see it.

But he said, "You have dipped your finger into the water. This time it may pass but take care you do not again let anything go in."

By daybreak the boy was already sitting by the well and watching it. His finger hurt him again. He passed it over his head and, unhappily, a hair fell into the well. He took it out quickly, but it was already gilded. Iron Hans came and already knew what had happened. "You have let a hair fall into the well," he said. "I will allow you to watch it once more, but if this happens for the third time, then the well is polluted and you can no longer remain with me."

On the third day, the boy sat by the well and did not stir his finger however much it hurt him. But the time was long to him, and he looked at the reflection of his face on the surface of the water. As he was doing so, bending over more and more and trying to look straight into the eyes, his long hair fell from his shoulders into the water. He raised himself quickly, but all the hair on his head was already golden

57

and shone like the sun. You can imagine how terrified the poor boy was! He took his pocket handkerchief and tied it round his head so that the man might not see it. But, when he came, he already knew everything and said, "Take off the handkerchief." Then the golden hair streamed out. Let the boy excuse himself as he might, it was no use. "You have not stood the trial and can stay here no longer. Go into the world; there you will learn what poverty is. But because you do not have a bad heart and I mean well by you, there is one thing I will grant you. If you fall into any difficulty, come to the forest and cry, "Iron Hans," and I will come and help you. My power is great—greater than you think, and I have gold and silver in abundance."

Then the king's son left the forest and walked by beaten and unbeaten paths ever onward until at length he reached a great city, where he looked for work, but could find none. He learned nothing by which he could help himself. Eventually, he went to the palace and asked if they would take him in. The people about court did not know what use they could make of him, but they liked him and told him to stay. Finally, the cook took him into his service and said he might carry wood and water and rake the cinders together.

Once, when no one else was at hand, the cook ordered him to carry the food to the royal table, but because he did not like for his golden hair to be seen, he kept his little cap on. Such a thing as that had not yet come to the king's notice and he said, "When you come to the royal table you must remove your hat."

He answered, "Ah, Lord, I cannot; I have a bad sore place on my head." With this, the king had the cook called before him and scolded him, asking how he could take such a boy into his service saying that he was to send him away at once. The cook, however, had pity on him and exchanged him for the gardener's boy.

Now the boy had to plant and water the garden, hoe and dig, and bear the wind and bad weather. Once in summer, when he was working alone in the garden, the day was so warm that he took his little cap off to let the air might cool him. As the sun shone on his hair, it glittered and flashed so that the rays fell into the bedroom of the king's daughter. Up she sprang to see what it could be. When she saw the boy, she cried to him, "Boy, bring me a wreath of flowers."

He put his cap on with haste, gathered wild field flowers, and bound them together. As he was ascending the stairs with them, the gardener met him and said, "How can you take the king's daughter a garland of such common flowers? Go quickly, and get another, and seek out the prettiest and rarest."

"Oh, no," replied the boy, "the wild ones have more scent and will please her more."

When he entered the room, the king's daughter said, "Take your cap off; it is not seemly to keep it on in my presence."

He said again, "I may not, I have a sore head." She, however, caught his cap and pulled it off. His golden hair rolled down onto his shoulders and was splendid to behold. He wanted to run away, but she held him by the arm and gave him a handful of ducats. With these he departed, but he cared nothing for the gold pieces. He took them to the gardener and said, "I present them to your children; they can play with them."

The following day the king's daughter again called to him to bring her a wreath of field flowers. When he went in with it, she instantly snatched at his cap and wanted to take it away from him, but he held it fast with both hands. She again gave him a handful of ducats, but he would not keep them and gave them to the gardener for his children's playthings. On the third day things went the same; she could not get his cap away from him, and he would not keep her money.

Not long after, the country was overrun by war. The king gathered his people and did not know whether he could offer any opposition to the enemy, who was superior in strength and had a mighty army. Then said the gardener's boy, "I am grown and will go to the war; just give me a horse."

The others laughed, and said, "Seek one for yourself when we are gone. We will leave one behind in the stable for you." When they had gone, he went into the stable and led the horse out. It was lame in one foot and limped hobblety jib, hobblety jib. Nevertheless, he mounted it and rode away to the dark forest. When he came to the outskirts, he called "Iron Hans" three times so loudly that it echoed through the trees.

With this, the wild man appeared immediately and said, "What do you desire?"

"I want a strong steed, for I am going to the war."

"That you shall have and still more than you ask." The wild man went back into the forest and it was not long before a groom emerged, leading a horse that snorted with its nostrils and could hardly be restrained. Behind them followed a great troop of warriors, equipped entirely in iron with swords flashing in the sunlight. The youth gave over his three-legged horse to the groom, mounted the other, and rode at the head of the soldiers.

When he got near the battlefield a great many of the king's men had already fallen and little wanted to make the rest give way. Then the youth galloped thither with his iron soldiers, broke like a hurricane over the enemy, and beat down all who opposed him. They began to flee, but the youth pursued and did not stop until not a single man was left.

Instead of returning to the king, however, he conducted his troops back to the forest and called Iron Hans.

"What do you desire?" asked the wild man. "Take back your horse and troops and give me my three-legged horse again." All that he asked was done and soon he was riding on his three-legged horse.

When the king returned to his palace, his daughter went to meet him and wished him joy for his victory. "I am not the one who carried the victory," he said, "but a strange knight who came to my assistance with his soldiers."

The daughter wanted to hear who the strange knight was, but the king did not know, and said, "He followed the enemy, and I did not see him again." She inquired of the gardener where his boy was, but he smiled and said, "He has just come home on his three-legged horse, and the others have been mocking him and crying, 'Here comes our hobblety jib back again!' They asked, too, 'Under what hedge have you been lying sleeping all the time?' So he said, 'I did the best of all, and it would have gone badly without me.' Then he was ridiculed even more."

The king said to his daughter, "I will proclaim a great feast that will last for three days, and you shall throw a golden apple. Perhaps the unknown man will show himself." When the feast was announced, the youth went out to the forest and called Iron Hans.

"What do you desire?" he asked.

"That I may catch the golden apple of the king's daughter."

"It is as good as if you had it already," said Iron Hans. "You shall likewise have a suit of red armor for the occasion and ride on a spirited chestnut horse."

When the day came, the youth galloped to the spot, took his place among the knights, and was recognized by no one. The king's daughter came forward and threw a golden apple to the knights, but none of caught it but he. But as soon as he had it, he galloped away.

On the second day, Iron Hans equipped him as a white knight and gave him a white horse. Again he was the only one who caught the apple, but did not linger an instant and galloped off with it.

The king grew angry and said, "This is not allowed; he must appear before me and tell his name." He gave the order that, if the knight who caught the apple should go away again, they should pursue him, and if he would not come back willingly, they were to cut him down and stab him.

On the third day, he received from Iron Hans a suit of black armor and a black horse. Again he caught the apple, but when he was riding off with it the king's attendants pursued him, and one of them got so near him that he wounded the youth's leg with the point of his sword. The youth nevertheless escaped from them, but his horse leapt so violently that the helmet fell from the youth's head and they could see that he had golden hair. They rode back and announced this to the king.

The following day the king's daughter asked the gardener about his boy. "He is at work in the garden; the strange creature has been at the festival, too, and came home only yesterday evening; he has likewise shown my children three golden apples that he won."

The king had him summoned to his presence, and he came again with his little cap on his head. The king's daughter went up to him and took it off, and his golden hair fell over his shoulders. He was so handsome that all were amazed. "Are you the knight who came every day to the festival, always in different colors, and who caught the three golden apples?" asked the king.

"Yes," he answered, "and here are the apples." He took them out of his pocket and returned them to the king. "If you desire further proof, you may see the wound that your people gave me when they followed me. I am likewise the knight who helped you to victory over your enemies."

"If you can perform such acts as that, you are no gardener's boy. Tell me, who is your father?"

"My father is a mighty king, and gold have I in plenty as great as I require."

"I well see," said the king, "that I owe my thanks to you. Can I do anything to please you?"

"Yes," he answered, "indeed you can. Give me your daughter to wife."

The maiden laughed, and said, "He does not stand much on ceremony, but I have already seen by his golden hair that he was no gardener's boy," and she went and kissed him.

His father and mother came to the wedding, and were in great delight, for they had given up all hope of ever seeing their dear son again. As they sat at the marriage feast, the music suddenly stopped, the doors opened, and a stately king came in with a great retinue. He went up to the youth, embraced him, and said, "I am Iron Hans, and was by enchantment a wild man, but you have set me free; all the treasures I possess shall be your property."[1]

~

It is obvious which metal process is described in the tale "Iron Hans."[2] The title itself announces it. No other fairy tale offers the key to understanding its imaginative language so clearly as this one. Iron is the earthly counterpart of the Mars sphere, which the "I" enters after leaving the Jupiter sphere on its incarnation journey. So in describing the iron process, we are at the same time grasping essential aspects of the Mars sphere.

The Essence of Iron

The essential qualities of iron are fittingly captured in the image of the knight encased in iron armor and bearing an iron sword. The armor grants him protection and security, while the sword enables him to test his mettle. Iron stands as an image for battle, courage and resolution, an aspect that is also expressed in its mythological association with Mars, the impetuous warrior deity. He appears among the gods fully armed and battle-ready. His attack is fearsome; his sharp sword conquers all resistance; hence he is known as the "invincible one."

Iron is also traditionally associated with the forceful, forward-marching choleric temperament. The word *choleric* itself refers to the bile, indicating the connection of this temperament with the gall bladder and its bile function. A flare of temper is connected with a surge of bile.

---

1   This version originally translated by E. Taylor (1905); http://etc.usf.edu /lit2go/175/grimms-fairy-tales/3177/iron-hans/ (revised).

2   A study of "Iron Hans" in light of the homeopathic remedy picture of iron was made by Martin Stübler. It is published in *Gold, Kupfer und Eisen aus der Sicht der Homöopathie und der durch Anthroposophie erweiterten Medizin*, Verga Editio, Krankenhaus Lahnhöhe, Koblenz, 1983. Paul Paede also interpreted "Iron Hans" from the viewpoint of the iron process. His study is published in the *Wochenschrift für Anthroposophie*, Goetheanum, Oct. 29, 1967, Dornach.

The Motifs of the Tale and the Iron Process

While the lead process is essentially past-oriented and the tin process is chiefly concerned with the present, the iron process is directed wholly toward the future. This is reflected in the forward-urging dynamic of the tale of Iron Hans. The past, even the king's son's own past, counts for little. He hides his golden hair to avoid revealing his royal descent, or past. How much simpler it would have been simply to reveal his princely identity! But for him, the present serves only as a way of shaping the future. At decisive moments the king's son always performs a courageous act that gives the plot a new twist.

The king's son grasps whatever opportunities appear to forge his destiny by his own power. This power, which makes him master of his future, can be described as the Mars dynamic. The Mars dynamic is always vigorously directed toward the goal; yet mere forward movement is not the main motif of "Iron Hans." Moving forward also always means overcoming resistance. The Mars dynamic needs obstacles to pit its strength against. This creates the field of tension in which growth and maturation can take place. The iron process wants resistance to purify itself; only in this way can it be "tempered."

Let us examine the process more closely. When the iron dynamic hits an obstacle, pressure and tension begin to build up. These modulate and structure its forward movement, giving rise to oscillation. A characteristic Mars organ is the larynx,[3] where the air stream builds pressure and comes to vibration, making possible to form speech. Living substance, protein, takes form in a similar way. In this case, the iron stream of the blood is "dammed up" in the liver. Within the field of tension of protein formation, iron mediates its structures to the liver.

As an aid to understanding such phenomena, Bernard Lievegoed pointed to the Chladni figures, which arise when a metal plate sprinkled with sand is brought into vibration using the bow of a stringed

---

3 Steiner, *At Home in the Universe,* Nov. 17, 1923, The Hague.

instrument. The sand forms fascinating patterns corresponding to the particular vibrations of the plate.

In much the same way the king's son is continually confronted with obstacles to overcome. When he has finally surmounted them, he is able to release Iron Hans from enchantment and gain his treasures. His success at these tests reveals his healthy iron nature. As a kitchen boy he is able to stand up to the king; as the gardener's boy he is able to control his passion for the princess; and as a knight he is able to defeat the enemy in battle. In fact, one may say that the tale imaginatively depicts three iron processes: those of the upper, the lower and the center poles of the human organization. We shall return to these later in more detail.

A series of images at the end of the tale allude to the iron-forging process. In its raw state, iron ore is red; in smelting it turns white; and hardened to steel its color is black. At the competition for the golden apple, the king's son appears first in red armor, then in white, and finally in black—pictures in which we can recognize the purification or tempering of the iron process represented by the king's son. These three colors depict the maturation of the iron forces in the human soul. The soul forces must pass through a stage of white heat or "steeling" before the individual can assume earthly power and exercise it with wisdom. This future prospect is conveyed in the fairy tale by the image of winning of the golden apples.

Thus the images of "Iron Hans" enable us to characterize the iron process generally as it acts in the human being. Now, as we examine specific images, we will discover that they can contribute to a detailed understanding of the iron dynamic.

The Iron Process and Human Development

The Iron Forces in Pregnancy and Childhood

The mood of iron is established right at the beginning of the tale with a courageous deed that sets the plot in motion. A daring hunter, ignoring all warnings, ventures into a dangerous wood where people and animals have been inexplicably disappearing. Fearlessly he enters the wood with his dog. As he watches a pool deep in the wood, a long arm reaches out of the water, seizes his dog and pulls it into the depths. Unshaken by this harrowing scene, the hunter keeps a cool head. He calls in helpers who empty the pool with buckets. It turns out that the arm belongs to a wild man who has hidden in the pond. Thus exposed, he is shackled and brought to the royal court, where he is held captive in a cage in the courtyard. The queen keeps the key to this cage under her pillow.

Let us contemplate these images from the perspective of iron. In the wild man hidden in the pool we can recognize the iron force at work in the human embryo as it grows in the womb. Just as the unborn child draws iron and other nutrients out of its mother, so the wild man pulls everything living into his pool. The emptying of the pool and exposing of the wild man to the sunlight can be interpreted as the process of birth. Then the iron force lies captive in a cage, while the queen keeps the key beneath her pillow. These images can be taken to indicate that after birth, the iron force is held back by the mother's soul forces. In early childhood the iron force cannot unfold fully but is bound to the mother relationship. Its action is still assumed by the mother, so to speak. This represents approximately the phase of childhood from birth up to the ninth year of life. Only then is there an initial separation from the mother, and the iron forces are set free. This is depicted in a marvelous way by the subsequent images of the tale.

The Iron Forces up to the Ninth Year of Life

As the king's son is playing with his golden ball in the courtyard, it rolls into the cage and falls into the hands of Iron Hans. To get his ball back, the young prince agrees to liberate him. He fetches the key from under his mother's pillow and unlocks the cage. In the process he pinches his finger in the door. Once Iron Hans has been freed, the young man is afraid of his parents and asks Iron Hans to take him along. Iron Hans withdraws to the wilderness and the king's son now lives there with him.

How can we interpret these images? The young prince playing with the golden ball indicates that some of his soul forces have been liberated. In all fairy tales, a golden ball or sphere represents soul forces still wholly in their pre-earthly, cosmic condition. They remain sun-like and golden through and through. These soul forces are now freed and fall into the power of the iron process. Under its sway they lose their innocence and cosmic connection. Their release from the mother bond is depicted in the images of the king's son fetching the key from under his mother's pillow, liberating Iron Hans and going off with him into the wilderness. The same developmental phase is described in "The Frog Prince," but from a completely different perspective. Here the golden ball falls into the well, where the frog takes possession of it. In this case it is not the progressive iron forces that seize the pure soul forces, but resistant ones that oppose development.

Let us also examine the motif of the finger a little more closely. It appears one other time in this tale, when the king's son is guarding the well for Iron Hans in the wilderness and his finger is gilded as he dips it in the water. This motif appears in other Grimms' tales as well. In "Hansel and Gretel," Hansel must hold out his finger to the witch so that she can feel if he has become fat enough to be eaten. In "The Seven Ravens," the sister cuts off her little finger and uses it as a key to open up the glass mountain, which eventually leads to the disenchantment of her brothers. Thus the motif of the finger always appears when a decisive change is in the offing; one development comes to an end and a new phase begins. The changes we are speaking of in this transitional phase of human development will be described in the section on "The Iron Process in the Human Biography."

The Iron Forces in Puberty

Iron Hans and the king's son (we are informed that he is eight years old when he leaves the royal court) now live in "the dark forest." Iron Hans sets the king's son the task of keeping watch over the gold well, which is as bright and clear as crystal. If anything were to fall into it, the well would be desecrated. Thus, day after day, the king's son sits at the edge of the well watching the crystal-clear water in which golden snakes and fishes swim. Once, his finger hurts so badly that, to cool it, he dips it into the water. Realizing that he has desecrated the well, he quickly draws his finger out, but too late; it has already turned golden. Iron Hans is lenient and tells him to resume his post watching over the well. Again his finger begins to hurt, and he brushes it over his head, causing a hair to fall into the water, and this too becomes golden. Again Iron Hans forgives the king's son, and he continues sitting at the well's edge. But time passes too slowly for him. Fascinated by his mirror image on the surface of the water, he wishes to look it in the eyes, and as he bends closer to the water all his hair falls into it. In horror he raises his head, but too late; his hair is already entirely golden. He attempts to conceal this with a kerchief, but Iron Hans is not fooled, and this time he is no longer willing to retain the king's son. He sends him out "into the world," saying that now he must learn what poverty is. Yet Iron Hans promises him that if he should ever come into difficulty, he will come to his aid. He need only call him.

Let us try to interpret these images. The motif of the well appears frequently in fairy tales. We must picture a deep well of traditional build. Such a well has many layers of meaning; it can be understood as an image for life itself or for the soul's inner experience.[4] In "Iron Hans," the well episode occurs at the moment when the young soul of the king's son becomes enmeshed in the iron forces and they begin to work freely in it. The soul forces now rise partially to consciousness. Their depths appear bottomless like the well, and they are still

4   Cooper, *An Illustrated Encyclopaedia of Traditional Symbols.*

pure. This purity is to be guarded. But the iron force that lives in the king's son wishes to unite itself with the depths of his soul. The iron type refuses to remain superficial. He wants to unite with the hidden depths of his own soul, for these provide the strength to develop as an individuality, as a complete human being.

Iron contains the forces that can unite the cosmos fully with the Earth and thus transform and redeem the earthly. At puberty, when physical maturity is reached, the iron forces are completely liberated. The soul forces feel drawn to the depths of their own being. In the fairy tale this is depicted in images of the king's son coming into contact with the gold well; first one finger, then one hair, and finally all the hair of his head are dipped in the water and turned to gold. The soul falls in love, as it were, with its physical image, its reflection in the water, and so is drawn down into the depths of the body. This is essentially a blinding, a self-deception that desecrates the soul. Yet in the process the King's son has now reached physical maturity and must go forth into the world. He must get to know poverty. Poverty, here, signifies the material world, the world that always appears limited and makes us keenly aware of our own lacks and limitations. Significantly, Iron Hans does not completely reject the king's son at this point, but promises to assist him in need, mentioning that he has "gold and silver in abundance." This gives an indication of the function of iron as unifier of Heaven and Earth. While the iron process thrusts the human being into the material world, into "poverty," the same process assures us of treasures of gold and silver when we need them—surely a reference to the spiritual world. The forces of iron work in both directions. They lend cosmic forces to the earthly, and they make it possible to fight for spiritual goals.

Now let us briefly reflect on what the image of the golden hair might signify. "Turning golden," in the context of this tale, indicates that the iron process now has a cosmic Sun connection. The king's son with golden hair becomes an image of the sacred warrior, the Warrior of God on Earth. When hair—the image of vitality and etheric forces—is golden (cf. also the chapter on "The Goose Girl"), it shows that the power of youth united with inner Sun forces has come to full expression.

Effectiveness through the Iron Forces

Proceeding with the tale, we see the king's son hire himself out as a cook at a castle. One day he is asked to carry the food to the king himself. He keeps on the cap which he wears to hide his golden hair. The king reproaches him for this, and by way of an excuse the "kitchen boy" answers that he must wear a cap because of sores on his head. Hereupon he is relieved of his kitchen duties and must work as gardener's help. He tends the plants in the castle garden. One day when the sun is very hot and he thinks himself alone, he takes off his cap. In the sunlight his golden hair glitters and flashes so "that the rays fell into the bedroom of the princess, and up she sprang to see what that could be." One senses an implicit inner connection here between the sun, the golden hair, and the bedroom of the princess. The princess summons the gardener and asks him to bring her flowers. The king's son brings her wildflowers of the field and she pulls off his cap to see his golden hair. The next two times, this game is repeated; the princess tries to take away his hat, but now he is on guard and she fails. She gives him ducats (money), yet he will not keep it for himself and gives it all to the gardener's children to play with. The implication of this entire episode is that when the iron force is rightly managed—the image of the king's son in the guise of a gardener—it gives us self-control in our feelings.

In the next phase of the tale the iron process reveals its full power but still does not allow itself to be recognized. Enemies invade the land. The gardener's boy wants to help in its defense and appeals to Iron Hans for a sturdy mount on which to set out for war. Iron Hans not only fulfills his request but gives him much more; a whole army fitted out in iron armament. With this force the king's son puts the enemy to flight, pursues and cuts them down them to the last man—no half-measures for the iron-type! Having crushed the enemy, the victorious hero returns his troops and his steed to Iron Hans and rides back to the castle on his limping old nag. No one seeing him imagines that he is the victor; only the princess has a suspicion. The others make fun of him and his wobbly horse.

In the merciless slaughter of the enemy, we have an image of the iron forces displaying their full efficacy when they meet resistance. It is the battle of self-assertion that is won through them. Of particular significance is not only the thoroughness and efficacy of the hero's deeds—not a man is left alive—but also his ability to rein in the iron power and not to be carried away by it. After his victorious self-assertion he is not in the least blinded by self-love and shows no interest in a hero's honors. Indeed, he does not even allow himself to be known for the victor, but returns inconspicuously to his old work. Nor is he bothered by the ridicule and scorn he faces.

The Winning of the Golden Apple

After this veritable "iron proving," the iron process enters a critical phase. A competition is proclaimed in which the princess casts a golden apple. If the apple can be seen as a symbol of earthly power,[5] then the golden apple symbolizes power over the earthly forces that is attained through maturity and exercised with wisdom. Three times the princess casts the golden apple. Each time the gardener's boy catches it and races off. Each time he appears in different armor and rides a different mount—the first time in red armor on a chestnut horse, the next in white armor on a white horse, and the third in black armor on a black horse. The colors reflect the previously mentioned metamorphosis of iron as it is processed; raw iron is red; heated it glows white; and as steel it turns black. Thus the three colors are an expression of a purification process, which we understand here as the metamorphosis of the iron process in the human organism. And the

---

5   The orb on the scepter of the Holy Roman Emperor was known as the *Reichsapfel,* "imperial apple" (TN).

image of the different-colored horses hints that this transformation also extends to the thought processes (cf. the chapter on tin). Only in this way can the king's son win the golden apples, marry the princess, and become king.

The Iron Process in the Human Biography

Let us examine the tale once more from the perspective of the iron process in the human being.[6] In magnificent images it illustrates the healthy iron forces as they work in the human being and the critical phases in human development as they relate to the iron force. According to our interpretation of the tale, it begins with a description of the iron process in the embryo. Here the iron forces are responsible for drawing the iron stream from the mother's organism into the fetus.

The fairy tale presents this in the image of Iron Hans dwelling in a deep pool and with his long arms drawing into the water everything living that dares come near. The draining of the pool is an image for birth. From birth until about the ninth year, the iron forces are tightly bound to the physical and cannot unfold in the child's soul life. In place of them, on the psychological plane it is the maternal forces that still shape the child's relation to the outer world.

At about the ninth year, the iron forces become free. This is a critical phase for the child. "I"-consciousness awakens, bringing the capacity for self-assertion. This liberation of soul forces is based on certain processes in the organism. The "I" takes hold of the metabolism in the lower pole, and in this way the higher "I" receives a lower counterpart with which it can enter into a reciprocal relationship. The iron forces play a crucial role in this process; and if this phase is disturbed, the child may easily feel overwhelmed and suffer from such symptoms as school headaches. The awakening of the iron forces on the soul plane and their release from the mother

---

6   Walter Holzapfel, "Das Eisen in der Hand des Schularztes," *Beiträge zu einer Erweiterung der Heilkunst* 3/4, 1954, Stuttgart.

connection are portrayed in the fairy tale as the liberation of Iron Hans from his cage. The engaging of the "I" in the lower metabolism is portrayed by the events at the well. The soul begins to unite itself with the depths of the organism. In the king's son's fascination with his reflection, and in the immersion of his hair in the gold well, aspects of the entry into puberty find expression.

Puberty has set in and young people are thrown upon their own resources. With the help of the iron forces, they must go out and find their way in the world, where they are confronted with various tests that challenge their iron forces. These are the tests of self-assertion, self-mastery, and self-realization. Self-assertion is connected with the upper pole of human beings; "cooks" keep a cap on their head; for now they live by their own thinking and ideas. Self-mastery—in this case mastering passions—has to do with the iron process in the middle sphere; "gardeners" keep their feelings for the princess in check. Self-realization, finally, is realized in the lower pole; "warriors" become knights and saviors. The enemy is a foreign power that would otherwise conquer and destroy them, and so they fight unconditionally.

The individuality is unable to integrate the three iron processes within itself until they have been truly mastered. The golden apples appear as a sign that this has been accomplished, symbolizing earthly power rightly exercised through wisdom, beauty, and goodness.

Disturbed Iron Processes

Now let us consider the fairy tale from the therapeutic point of view. It portrays the healthy iron process as it acts in normal human development. By replacing the images of the tale with their opposites we can recognize the disease pictures for which iron is therapeutically effective. There are two disease pictures associated with a disturbed, uncontrolled iron process. First is the picture of obvious weakness in the iron process; then there is a picture which may be in part an overcompensation; the patient displays the outward symptoms of an excessive iron process, but these are in fact based on a weak, uncontrolled iron process.

Unlike the other planetary metals, iron occurs substantially in the organism. In the case of the other metals—gold or lead, for example—only the metal *process* is active in the organism. With iron, the *substance itself* carries out important functions in the organism. This may be the reason that there is essentially no such thing as an excessive iron process in the organism.

Even in the healthy organism iron is present in excess, so in this sense no intensification is possible. When disease pictures indicate an excessive iron process, the patient's weakness is an inability to control it, not an overly strong process itself. For this reason, with very few exceptions iron preparations are given in low potencies or wholly unpotentized. High potencies, which counteract an excessive process in other metals, are rarely used with iron.

The Disturbed Iron Process in the Nerve-Sense System

To repeat, the first test in this tale is one of self-assertion. Self-assertion requires a healthy self-confidence. If this is given, one is largely freed of the need for outward recognition and can accept humiliations unperturbed. This is the attitude we find in the king's son when he hires himself out as a kitchen boy at the castle. A disturbed iron process, on the other hand, may find expression in anxiety, passivity, faintheartedness, indecisiveness, apathy and withdrawal. In the case when the iron process is adequate but uncontrolled, however, the patient may display aggression, self-inflation, and a craving for recognition and affirmation. Both pictures reflect a fundamental lack of self-confidence, which in the second case patients generally do not admit to themselves.

The therapy includes various iron preparations that have a relation to the iron process and/or the nerve-sense system. Thus for insecurity and anxiety, the iron-arsenic compound *Scorodite* (*Skorodit* D10) has proven effective.

On the functional plane low self-confidence, i.e., insufficient psychic stability, is expressed in vascular lability and vascular erethism. This can be quite problematic for young people so affected. They feel "caught out" or seen through, and with a sudden rush of blood to the head they blush uncontrollably. They lack the composure to deal with an unpleasant situation.

The Disturbed Iron Process in the Rhythmic System[7]

Now let us move on to the middle iron process, beginning again with the related fairy-tale images. The king's son now works as a gardener, tending the plant kingdom. Plants embody the middle iron process. The iron in the green chlorophyll of the leaves stands between the "heavenly iron" of the meteorites and the specifically earthly iron element of the ores, and so has a mediating function between above and below. The princess is dazzled by the radiance of the gardener's golden hair. A passion is developing, one that the princess for her part openly reveals. The king's son, however, masters his emotions completely. These images reflect the vital, healthy iron process of the middle sphere. People with a well-developed iron process in the middle sphere generally demonstrate the qualities of prudence, presence of mind, and bravery in difficult situations. In exceptional cases this can extend to the highest degree of personal courage—risking or sacrificing one's own life for others. History offers us abundant examples of this level of the purified, mastered iron process.

When the middle iron process is disturbed, on the other hand, affection for another human being can erupt as an uncontrolled passion. The connection becomes emotionally overcharged and unrealistic. The patient shows exaggerated self-reference in his relations with others. Ego takes hold of the feeling life. This disturbance in

---

7   Karl König, "Der dreifache Eisenprozeß," *Beiträge zu einer Erweiterung der Heilkunst* 9/10, 1950–51, Stuttgart; Olaf Titze, "Zur Frage der Wirkungsrichtungen von verschiedenen Klassen der Mineralien am Beispiel der Eisenverbindungen," *Mitteilungen der wissenschaftlichen Mitarbeiter der Weleda AG*, Jahresinformationstagung in Schwäbisch Gmünd, 1982.

the patients' relationships to those close to them can be expressed in various disease pictures. One such image is hysteria, which can be treated with *Katoptrite* (*Katoptrit* D6), a compound of iron and antimony. *Katoptrite* stimulates the iron process to resume its wholesome mediating function between the upper and lower poles.

The Disturbed Iron Process in the Metabolic System

The lower iron process is reflected in the deeds of the king's son as the warrior—the hero who not only routs the enemy but pursues and destroys them utterly. This is a clear example the choleric element that is never willing to stop until the job is completely done. The physiological counterpart of this description is the bile function. Bile attacks the nutrient stream as a foreign element entering the organism and overcomes it. The foreign nature of food is conquered to the very last particle. Only then can food be absorbed into the organism. The bile process is one of self-assertion for the organism, enabling it to realize its selfhood. This creates the physical "self-space." The bile process, with which the choleric element is associated, is also a will process and always therefore requires activity.

A disturbance of the lower iron process can manifest itself in two directions. A strong but uncontrolled iron process is seen frequently in daredevil or hothead types who are drawn to wild, explosive behavior. A deficient iron process, in contrast, can be seen in the lethargic, the weak, and the cowardly who are unable to stand up for themselves. The excessive process produces overstimulation, sudden rage, time pressure, and mania; the deficient one is reflected in flagging energy, resentment, and cholagenic (bile-related) depression.

When a disturbance of the metabolic iron process manifests in liver and gallbladder dysfunction, the chief preparations indicated are *Ferrum metallicum, Ferrum sulfuratum,* and *Siderit* in low potencies. On the other hand, if the disturbed iron process is connected with deficient "kidney radiation," thus creating generalized weakness and hypotonia, then *Solutio ferri* is frequently helpful. If the weakness is the result of a recent flu, for example, then *Ferrum sidereum* D6 is frequently prescribed.

Iron Hans as Warrior of God on Earth

After the events in the tale that we have described as the lower iron processes, the king's son wins the golden apple three times in a row, marries the princess and frees Iron Hans from enchantment. He has attained maturity as a human being and mastery of the earthly plane. Yet this is not mastery in the usual sense—that of exercising power—but the ability to conduct his life with wisdom and righteousness. The goldenness of the apple shows that the divine realm has now been incorporated. Reversing this picture to find the therapeutic applications of iron, we see that when the iron process is disturbed the earthly plane cannot be mastered in harmony. It will not be possible to win the golden apple, that is, to act on Earth as a warrior for the good and just. The patient has lost his cosmic connection and the spiritual source of power for his actions. Either he is at the mercy of his own uncontrolled temperament, or he is simply too weak to engage effectively in the world.

Now we come to the end of the tale. When the king's son wins the third golden apple and rushes off the field for the third time, a servant of the king manages to catch up with him and wound him in the leg. The king's son's horse rears so violently that he loses his helmet and reveals his golden hair. Now it is obvious to all who the unknown knight is. He is called before the king and reveals himself as the son of a rich and mighty king. The king feels indebted to him and gladly assents when the prince asks for his daughter's hand. Among the guests at the wedding are his parents and a stately king who arrives with a great retinue. He approaches the youth, embraces him and announces, "I am Iron Hans. I was by enchantment a wild man, but you have redeemed me. All the treasures I possess shall be yours."

The course of events depicted in these magnificent images demonstrates to us how iron as a cosmic principle can be made serviceable for the earthly human life. Such a person can rightly be called a Warrior of God.[8] Now the iron process has purified its martial, earthly nature. The vehement, untamed, egoistic element of the process has been overcome and it rises to a new unity—one that embraces the feminine aspect of cosmic wisdom as well. Therefore the young king not only receives the princess as his spouse, but the "treasures of Iron Hans" also belong to him. In other words, purified, "golden" heart forces embracing all existence are now available to him without limitation.

---

8   This suggests the image of Michael, the archangel who has the power to put cosmic iron to his service. (Steiner, *At Home in the Universe*, Nov. 17, 1923, The Hague.)

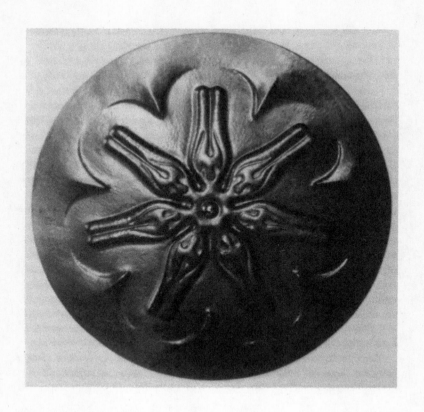

Mars Seal

Gold as a Remedy: "Hans in Luck"

Hans had served his master as an apprentice for seven years, and so he said to him, "Master, my time is up. Now I would like to go back home to my mother. Give me my wages."

The master answered, "You have served me faithfully and honestly. As the service was, so shall the reward be." And he gave Hans a piece of gold as big as his head.

Hans pulled his handkerchief out of his pocket, wrapped up the lump in it, put it on his shoulder, and set out on the way home. As he went on, always putting one leg before the other, he saw a horseman trotting quickly and merrily by on a lively horse. "Ah," said Hans quite loudly, "what a fine thing it must be to ride. There you sit as on a chair, never stumbling over a stone, saving your shoes, and making your way without even knowing it."

The rider heard him. He stopped and called out, "Hey there, Hans, then why are you traveling on foot?"

"I must," answered Hans, "for I have this lump to carry home. It is true that it is gold, but I cannot hold my head straight for it, and it hurts my shoulders."

"I'll tell you what," said the rider. "Let's trade. I will give you my horse, and you can give me your lump of gold."

"With all my heart," said Hans. "But I can tell you that you will be dragging along with it."

The rider got down, took the gold and helped Hans up and gave him the bridle tight in his hands and said, "If you want to go fast, you must click your tongue and call out, 'Gee-up.'"

Hans was heartily delighted as he sat on the horse and rode away bold and free. After a while he thought that it ought to go faster and began to click with his tongue and call out, "Gee-up." The horse started a fast trot, and before Hans knew where he was, he was thrown off and lying in a ditch that separated the fields from the highway. The horse would have escaped if it had not been stopped by a peasant, who was coming along the road herding a cow before him.

Hans pulled himself together and stood up, but he was vexed and said to the peasant, "It is a poor joke, this riding, especially when I get hold of a mare like this that kicks and throws me off, so that I might break my neck. I will never mount it again. I like your cow. I could walk quietly behind her and always have my milk, butter, and cheese each day. What would I not give to have such a cow?"

"Well," said the peasant, "if it would give you so much pleasure, I do not mind trading the cow for the horse." Hans agreed with great delight, and the peasant jumped on the horse and rode away.

Hans drove his cow quietly before him and thought about his lucky bargain. "If only I had a morsel of bread—and that can hardly fail me—I could eat butter and cheese with it as often as I like. If I am thirsty, I can milk my cow and drink the milk. My goodness, what more could I possibly want?"

Finally, he arrived at an inn and stopped. To celebrate his good fortune, he ate everything he had with him, his dinner, supper, and all he had and, with his last few farthings, had half a glass of beer. Then he drove his cow on in the direction of his mother's village.

As noon approached, the heat grew oppressive, and Hans found himself on a moor that would take at least another hour to cross. He felt very hot, and his tongue stuck to the roof of his mouth with thirst. "I can find a cure for this," thought Hans. "I will milk the cow now and refresh myself with the milk." He tied her to a withered tree and, as he had no pail, put his leather cap underneath. But try as he might, not a drop of milk came. Because he was working in a clumsy way, the impatient beast finally gave him such a blow on the head with its hind foot that he fell to the ground and did not know where he was for a long time.

By good fortune, a butcher then came along the road with a push-cart in which a young pig lay. "What sort of a trick is this?" he cried, and helped poor old Hans up. Hans told him what had happened. The butcher gave him his flask and said, "Take a drink and refresh yourself. The cow will certainly give no milk. It is an old beast. At best, it is fit only for the plow or for the butcher."

"Well, well," said Hans, as he stroked his hair down on his head. "Who would have thought it? Certainly it is a fine thing when one can slaughter a beast like that for oneself. What meat one has! But I do not care much for beef, it is not juicy enough for me. But to have a young pig like that! It tastes quite different, and there are sausages, as well."

"Listen, Hans," said the butcher. "To do you a favor, I will trade and let you have the pig for the cow."

"God reward you for your kindness," said Hans as he gave up the cow. The pig was untied from the cart, and the cord by which it was tied was put in his hand, and Hans went on, thinking to himself how everything was going just as he wished. If anything troublesome happened to him, it was immediately set right.

Presently he was joined by a lad carrying a fine white goose under his arm. They greeted each other and Hans began to tell of his good luck and how he had always made such good trades. The boy told him that he was taking the goose to a christening feast. "Just heft her," he added, taking hold of her by the wings. "Feel how heavy she is. She has been fattened up for the last eight weeks. Anyone who bites into her after she has been roasted will have to wipe the fat from both sides of his mouth."

"Yes," said Hans, hefting her with one hand, "she weighs a lot, but my pig is not so bad either."

Meanwhile the lad looked suspiciously from one side to the other and shook his head. "Look here," he said at last. "It may not be all right with your pig. In the village I passed through, the mayor himself had just had one stolen out of its sty. I fear that you have hold of it there. They have sent out some people, and it would be a bad business if they caught you with the pig. At the very least, you would be shut up in the dark hole."

Poor Hans was terrified. "For goodness' sake," he said, "help me out of this fix. You know more about this place than I do. Take my pig and leave me your goose."

"I am taking a risk," answered the lad, "but I do not want to be the cause of your getting into trouble." So he took the cord in his hand and quickly drove the pig down a side path.

Hans, freed from care, headed toward home with the goose under his arm. "When I think about it properly," he said to himself, "I have even gained by the trade. First there is the good roast meat, then the quantity of fat that will drip from it and give me goose fat for my bread for a quarter of a year, and finally the beautiful white feathers. I will have my pillow stuffed with them, and then indeed I shall go to sleep without being rocked. How glad my mother will be!"

As he was going through the last village, there stood a scissors grinder with his cart as his wheel whirred he sang, "I sharpen scissors and quickly grind, my coat blows out in the wind behind."

Hans stood and looked at him. At last he said to him, "All's well with you, as you are so merry with your grinding."

"Yes," answered the scissors grinder, "this trade has a golden foundation. A real grinder is a man who as often as he puts his hand into his pocket finds gold there. But where did you buy that fine goose?"

"I did not buy it, but traded my pig for it."

"And the pig?"

"I got it for a cow."

"And the cow?"

"I got it for a horse."

"And the horse?"

"For that I gave a lump of gold as big as my head."

"And the gold?"

"Well, that was my wages for seven years' service."

"You have known how to look after yourself each time," said the grinder. "If you can only get to the point where you hear money jingle in your pocket whenever you stand up, you will have made your fortune."

"How will I manage that?" said Hans.

"You must become a grinder, as I am. Nothing particular is needed for it but a grindstone. Everything else takes care of itself. I have one here. It is certainly a little worn, but you need not give me anything for it but your goose. Will you do it?"

"How can you ask?" answered Hans. "I shall be the luckiest fellow on Earth. If I have money whenever I put my hand in my pocket, why should I ever worry again?" And he handed him the goose and received the grindstone in exchange.

"Now," said the grinder, picking up an ordinary heavy stone that lay nearby, "here is another good stone for you as well, which you can use to hammer on and straighten your old nails. Carry it along with you and take good care of it."

Hans loaded himself with the stones and went on with a contented heart, his eyes shining with joy. "I must have been born with lucky skin," he cried. "Everything I want happens to me just as if I were a Sunday's child." Meanwhile, as he had been on his legs since daybreak, he began to feel tired. Hunger also tormented him, for in his joy at the bargain by which he got the cow he had eaten up all his store of food at once. Finally he could continue only with great difficulty and was forced to stop every minute.

The stones, too, weighed him down, and he could not help thinking how nice it would be if he would not have to carry them just then. He crept along like a snail until he came to a well in a field, where he thought that he would rest and refresh himself with a cool drink of water. Too avoid damaging the stones while sitting down, he placed them carefully by his side at the edge of the well. Then he sat on it and was about to lean over to drink when he slipped, pushed against the stones, and both of them fell into the water. When Hans saw them sinking to the bottom with his own eyes, he jumped for joy and then knelt and, with tears in his eyes, thanked God for having shown him this favor, too, and delivered him in so good a way and without his having any need to reproach himself, from those heavy stones that had been the only things troubling him.

"No one under the sun is as fortunate as I am," he cried out. With a light heart and free from every burden he now ran on until he was at home with his mother.[1]

The Essence of Gold

Gold is a metal that exercises a special fascination over human beings. The possession of gold signifies riches, even power, and enhances our sense of self-worth in a special way. We adorn ourselves with it to underscore our personal value. Especially remarkable is the place occupied by gold in economic life; to this day it remains the measure of monetary value, and as a "hard" reserve it underpins our financial stability. It is laboriously brought up from the depths of the Earth, only to be deposited again in the underground vaults of the great banks. This material aspect has a power over human beings that can be described with no other term than "magical"; but alongside of it gold exhibits another, quite different and positive side; it is, and has always been, the metal of which ritual objects, ritual garments, insignias, and holy images are fashioned. The classic example of a gold culture in this sense was that of the Incas in the Andes, where gold could never be the property of a person but only of the gods. It could be used only by initiates, priests, and kings. Here we recognize the spiritual side of gold.

Regarding the relation of the spiritual to the material side of gold, Friedrich Benesch writes, "From its originally spiritual and divine past, gold has fallen into all kinds of demonic abysses. It

---

1   From english-magazine.org/index.php/english-stories/670-lucky-hans
     -english-story-of-the-month-april (revised).

bears today the curse that the dwarf Alberich laid on the gold of the Rhine daughters in the Nibelungen Saga. Gold comes into the possession of the dragon. Wisdom and Sun-filled will are overpowered by egoism and lust for power and possessions. Gold passes from hand to hand, but it is a treacherous possession. It grants not only wisdom in service of the gods, but also a darkening of our humanity in the service of matter."[2]

Thus, materialization and spiritualization are the two poles of gold and of the gold process. According to Rudolf Steiner, the entire spiritual and material cosmos is held in balance by the gold process.[3] In man as the microcosm, gold affects not only the mental and emotional life—the soul life—but as a process it also affects the bodily functions. The heart in particular is the organ through which it expresses its nature. In the systole its action is contracting, in the diastole expanding. Systole can be regarded as the process of incarnation and materialization, diastole as that of excarnation and spiritualization. These polarities are held in balance by the gold process.

In regard to gold as a substance, it should be added that it is the purest metal. It is practically indestructible and imperishable; it wishes to be only itself. For this reason the alchemists of the Middle Ages saw gold as the metal in which the three principles of "sal," "mercury," and "sulphur" are most intimately united.[4] This view explained to them the special properties of gold.

The Motifs of "Hans in Luck" and the Gold Process

The Grimms' "Hans in Luck" casts light on the various aspects of the gold process and the therapeutic use of gold in anthroposophic and homeopathic medicine. Looking first at the mood of the story, we recognize in it the sun quality of the gold process. The tale evokes a feeling of lightheartedness. Nothing really bad happens; everything

---

2   Benesch, *Apokalypse.*

3   Steiner, *Introducing Anthroposophical Medicine,* Mar. 26, 1920, Dornach.

4   Ibid.

is bathed in good cheer and brightness. As we follow the protagonist Hans-in-Luck, an image of the "Sun type" takes form. The Sun type can be described as openhearted, trusting, natural, generous, and self-confident, and this character description fits Hans-in-Luck perfectly. His optimistic attitude toward life, taking from each misadventure only its positive side, is that of a Sun nature.

In its main motif, the tale tells of how a heavy lump of pure gold is lost—how through a series of exchanges this valuable possession is traded for other goods of ever lower value until in the end Hans is entirely divested of possessions. A sad story? No, for now he can run home to his mother, free and light of heart. If we interpret the loss of possessions and the gaining of a joyful heart as the path of spiritualization, then this tale points to the essence of the gold process. Let us look into this more deeply.

The Gold Process and the Path to the Self

The plot of "Hans in Luck" is based on a seeming paradox. As wages for seven years of faithful work Hans receives a lump of gold "as big as his head"—a significant image in itself, by the way. In the five successive transactions—the gold for a horse, the horse for a cow, the cow for a pig, the pig for a goose, and the goose for a grindstone— he loses his entire earnings. Yet far from being downcast or unhappy, with each exchange right down to the ultimate loss of the grindstone, Hans feels a mounting sense of good fortune. And in the end, when there is nothing left of his wages, he thanks God for so mercifully freeing him from his last burden. This strikes the reader as an odd reaction; after all, most of us would be vexed at the loss of a lump of gold. But the tale has a truth to tell, so let us try to plumb it.

The entire action of the tale takes place in broad daylight. The sun is shining; in fact, at times the heat is oppressive. For a time Hans' homeward journey takes him across a moor where there is hardly any shade, as no trees or bushes grow there. Though he suffers from thirst, Hans does not encounter any truly threatening powers; the forces of Evil do not challenge him; no witch enchants him. It is also noteworthy that only Hans' homeward journey figures in the tale. He does not first set out into the wide world as in other fairy tales; from the very start he is only on the way home. Hans wends his way home through a landscape flooded with light and warmth.

What is the tale telling us when it says that Hans is on the way "home to his mother"? He is traveling the path that leads to himself; and the way to the self is a path of renunciation. In vivid images we are confronted with the paradox that through self-surrender and selflessness, the eternal nature of the human entelechy, the "I," can be found. This is also the path that leads to the heart, which is why in the end Hans is able to jump up with a light heart, free of all burdens, and run home to his mother—and why, at the end, he is able to exult, "There is no one under the sun so fortunate as I." The shining sun in the sky and the light heart in the human breast; this is the correspondence that matters at the end of the path. Hans has walked the sun path that leads to the heart, the organ of the higher Self, the "I."

The Sun Type

It is the gold process that makes this path possible for the human being; and as its personification, Hans-in-Luck presents a fully articulated picture of the gold process. If the merry happenings of this tale were turned upside down, it would show the disease picture for which gold is used therapeutically. This fact offers empirical confirmation that the tale refers to the gold process. Later we shall return to the therapeutic aspects of the remedy Aurum; here let us get a picture of the healthy gold process as the tale portrays it in the person of Hans.

Illustrations of this tale created by contemporaries of the brothers Grimm portray a Hans-in-Luck of medium-height or even on the short side and tending toward pyknic constitution,[5] but with a natural, upright posture. His face appears evenly formed, oval to round,

---

5   Of short and stocky physique (TN).

his skin rosy, his expression generous. As a Sun type Hans possesses large lively eyes that take in everything around him. We sense that the bloods pulses warm and strong through his veins. His character is so pure as to appear simple-minded, but he acts with confidence. As a Sun nature he knows no enemies but bears benevolence toward all he meets and believes the best of everyone. He accepts disappointments without embitterment and quickly forgets injustices done to him. Like the spring sunlight that calls the plant world to life, he enlivens the seeds of future possibilities through his affirming warmth. Faith, trust, and life-affirmation lie in his nature. Whatever new thing enters his field of vision he meets with benevolent interest. As an extrovert he is quickly roused to enthusiasm for something new, but if it proves unworthy he can let go of it just as quickly, completely freeing himself of it inwardly. The dominant polarity of his character is clearly that of taking hold and letting go—a contraction and expansion like the systole and diastole of the heart.

The Seven Steps to Selflessness

Through a sequence of seven steps, Hans-in-Luck attains selflessness. After that he desires nothing more for himself and thanks God for his merciful deliverance from the burdens of the Earth. Six of the seven steps entail a loss; the gold, the horse, the cow, the pig, the goose, and the grindstone—all are lost. And what is gained in return? Nothing—that is, the state of release. Yet this is a selflessness that Hans did not possess from the beginning. He was not bashful in requesting the wages for his seven years of labor, even though they posed a heavy load. And when he saw the horseman, his feelings were hardly pure; he was jealous of him for his effortless way of traveling. But with each further exchange his desire for the new possession weakens. Each new acquisition is connected with a certain trial. He fails to master the lively horse; and when it has thrown him, he sees the advantages of a quiet and useful cow. But his vain attempts to get milk from her are rewarded with a kick to the head that sends him sprawling. With the pig he finds he may even be accused of theft, and so the chance to exchange it for a goose appears as a salvation to him. He has now learned caution, and before the final exchange with the scissors grinder, he takes his time and looks at him before addressing him. What he receives in this transaction is merely a damaged stone of no value... and a new burden. Only when the heavy stone is resting at the bottom of the well is Hans' soul cleansed of desires and possessiveness. Now his heart is light.

Amusing as these exchanges may be, they are images for stages on the path of purification on which the soul must let go of all earthly values. This is the soul's journey to inwardness, to mystical entrance into its own spiritual nature, to its spiritual home. With the fall of the stone into the well, the earthly "I" has plumbed the unconscious depths of the soul, there to undergo mystical transfiguration.

Let us examine more carefully each step on the way to selflessness and to selfhood depicted in the tale.

The Horse

To review the relevant elements of this episode, Hans is walking along with his heavy lump when a horseman comes riding his way. He is captivated by the apparent ease of this mode of transportation, imagining he could ride just as well as the horseman if only he had a horse. In a moment they have struck a bargain: Hans surrenders his gold and receives the horse in return. Free of care he rides on for a time, but when his progress seems too slow, he clicks his tongue and calls "giddy up." The horse goes into a trot, and before Hans knows what has happened finds himself sprawled out in a ditch, dazed.

If this episode is taken as an imaginative depiction of a soul process, then Hans is—literally—"getting up on his high horse." His wish is to be carried along effortlessly, to have a "free ride." It is a kind of arrogance. His fantasy, however, comes to an abrupt end as the inexperienced rider lands on Earth—in fact a bit lower, in the ditch. Thus the first stage of the way can be understood as a purging of arrogance, of conceit, of the desire to occupy a higher position than one deserves and to get along more quickly than the pedestrians. One is reminded here of the automobile, which serves not just the practical purpose of transportation but so often also is an object of prestige for that part of us which needs external confirmation.

The Cow

The next scenes of the tale present a counter-image to the first stage of the way. After his fall, Hans has exchanged his horse for a cow. What appeals to him in the cow is that one can take one's time walking behind it, as well as the milk and butter and cheese it will give. What Hans sees in the cow is comfort and ease. In fact, the very next thing he does is to stop at an inn, eat up all of his remaining provisions and spend the last of his money on a half glass of beer. He is out to enjoy life to the full. But his greed leads to a bad outcome too when he is kicked, knocked to the ground and unable to recall where he is. The lesson of this second episode might be formulated thus: When self-indulgent dreams of enjoyment and high living run up against their physical limits, the awakening is brutal and thorough.

The Pig

A butcher carrying a young pig in a wheelbarrow "by chance" crosses Hans' path. Again an exchange is made and Hans is overjoyed at the solution to his problems. His mind conjures up images of the juicy pork and sausages he will get when it is slaughtered. But troubles of a new and special kind arise when a lad carrying a pretty white goose under his arm joins him and insinuates that something "may not be quite right" with this pig, that it was stolen and that Hans would be "shut up in the dark hole" if he were caught with it. So now, beset by fear and anxiety, Hans exchanges the pig for the goose with this helpful lad who is only too glad to relieve him of his pig. The exchange completed, Hans resumes his homeward journey free of cares.

In the first two phases of Hans' journey home—as a rider whose arrogance takes a fall and as a cowherd whose gluttony comes to an abrupt end—we see descriptions of particular imbalances of the *Aurum* patient. Here are character traits formed by the gold process in an unbalanced and therefore unhealthy way. Tendencies toward both arrogance and lavish living frequently appear in this type. Before we consider this further, let us look into the meaning of the images in the pig episode.

The pig is an animal with a very labile circulation. Under stress it is prone to circulatory collapse, and any excitement drives its blood pressure up and stresses the heart. Whatever influences the soul life of this animal is transmitted directly to the circulation. In its perceptual life the pig is completely bound to the sense-world. This is what lies behind the German insult *du armes Schwein* (roughly, "you miserable swine")—part pity, part contempt. The pig is a symbol of bondage to the material world with all its limitations; it can experience only the "lower" side of existence. In this condition the soul may feel as though shut up in a dark prison. It is not a coincidence that feelings of anxiety are connected in this tale with the pig. Because of the pig, Hans must fear being shut up in a dark and narrow place from which there is no escape. This is a description that quite frequently applies to the soul world of *Aurum* patients when the first symptoms of pathology appear in the circulation.

The Goose

Hans, as the representative of the human being on the path of development, has rid his soul of traits of arrogance, indulgence in high living, and enchainment to the sensory world. Now he is ready to move on to finding himself, his "I."

Hans has certainly been rescued from a tight spot by trading the pig for a goose, but he has yet to recognize the benefits of this transaction. With the previous trades, the motivation always came from him, but now for the first time he agrees to a deal that brings him no obvious benefit. Before too long, however, he begins to see positive sides of this exchange too. He pictures a nice roasted goose, goose fat for his bread, soft white feathers for a pillow on which he imagines "going to sleep without rocking." Thus, with the acquisition of the goose Hans has regained his inner equilibrium. His mind has become calm enough to entertain the idea of blissful sleep.

Acquiring the goose is connected with Hans' ability to regain peace within and harmony with the world. Ancient traditions connect the goose with the power of the Sun. The shape of this well-fed bird seems to have appeared as an embodiment of stored solar energy. The tradition of serving roast goose at Martinmass or Christmas was not just a matter of feasting; it expressed the idea that the Sun's light had come to human beings in physical form, and that everyone could partake of it. In more general terms, the goose is a symbol of life- and growth-giving warmth. Geese have also always been connected with special capacities of the soul—watchfulness and wakefulness—as we are reminded by the Roman legend of the Capitoline geese.[6]

The Grindstone

After he has passed the last village, Hans meets a scissors-grinder. For a long time he watches the man turning his wheel and cheerfully singing, but says not a word himself. He has become reticent. At the beginning of his travels he expressed his every feeling in words and gestures; now he looks on quietly. At last Hans recounts the steps of his adventures; then he is ready for the last exchange—the goose for a damaged grindstone! Out of the goodness of his heart the scissors-grinder gives him a bonus—an ordinary stone that "you can hammer

---

6   According to this legend, the sacred geese of Juno alerted the guard atop the Capitoline hill of Rome to an approaching band of Gauls, who had climbed so stealthily that not even the dogs noticed them (TN).

well upon." Contented, Hans resumes his journey carrying his heavy stones. But very quickly he becomes tired from the long day's march and can hardly go on without stopping to rest every moment. The stones press hard on his shoulders and it occurs to him how happy he would be to be rid of them. He slowly drags himself to a well where he can rest and refresh himself with a drink. He sets the stones carefully on the rim of the well, but as he bends over to drink, he knocks them in and they sink to the bottom.

By connecting himself with the goose, Hans has become ready to take the last remaining step before he can really come "home to his mother," his spiritual source. He takes up two stones, one of which is a grindstone. The special thing about a grindstone is that in the process of sharpening it emits a shower of sparks, almost a fire; the stone reveals its fiery inner life. The Old Testament gives us a picture of stone in its purified form as a symbol of divine power. Sleeping on a stone, Jacob dreams of a ladder to Heaven and recognizes this stone as the House of God, Beth-El. And the mystic Hildegard von Bingen addresses God as "Thou high stone."

To carry "stones home on one's shoulders" is to carry one's "touchstone," one's uniquely individual "cross." It is an event specific to each human being. Hence acquiring the spark-casting grindstone can be seen as a sign that divine fire has struck in the soul and made it sparkle. And when in the end the stones fall into the well and disappear in the depths of the water, this suggests that the divine fire has become one with the human soul. The well always signifies a source of life for the human being; here, it stands for the soul that is receptive to spiritual knowledge. So through this last image the tale depicts Hans's newfound ability, as by an act of grace, to unite himself totally with the divine-spiritual in his soul. This is redemption, mystical union with God; and it is fitting to be thankful for it with tears in one's eyes. In this light it is also understandable that Hans ran on "with a light heart and free from every burden... until he was with his mother at home."

The *Aurum* Patient

This path of purification of the heart is made possible by the healthy gold process. An imbalanced *Aurum* process, as mentioned above, promotes pathological processes that are recognizable as reversals of the fairy-tale images. Such conditions benefit from gold in potentized form, since the body's inherent gold process can be stimulated to ordered activity by the remedy *Aurum*. Therefore by describing the disease pictures that are cured with potentized *Aurum*, we are giving a picture of the dynamic of gold in the human being. At the same time new aspects of the Hans-in-Luck's purification path come to light.

For a character typology of the *Aurum* patient, we must reverse our description of Han's character. The antithesis of this "pure fool," who always seems to act to his self-detriment, are the successful and dynamic managers of today's business world. These are people who always look to their own and their firm's advantage in their dealings. They are ruthless and pushy and "capitalize" on every situation. They must always be ready to pounce to avoid missing opportunities, and when that happens they lose sleep over it. They are also hard workers, steaming with energy to get things done. Their sight is set on achieving higher positions that bring respect. Thus, they become CEOs of organizations, sit on various administrative councils, and throw themselves into countless initiatives. They take the floor in all discussions and know how to drive home a point using emphatic rhetoric and powerful gestures. They always know exactly what they want and how to reach their goals—visible, tangible, earthly "gold." Tending toward the choleric by temperament, at the slightest contradiction they fly into a rage and display complete intolerance of differing views and opinions. Such a soul has a strong worldly orientation. They love fine cuisine; like to be known as wine connoisseurs; dress fashionably but unostentatiously; are seen at the wheel of cars befitting their rank; value the ambiance of luxury hotels; and so on. In short, they "love life" and see themselves as the unquestioned center. Yet it is really only themselves that they love.

It is not difficult to see certain connections between such a character and Hans-in-Luck, although outwardly they stand at opposite poles. From the viewpoint of the business world, Hans is of course the dropout, the loser, and the successful careerist is the winner. Yet careerists, precisely because of their activities, are rarely able to find their own self; in the final analysis, they are really the ones who come up empty. The reason this is worth examining is that it helps us understand the disease picture for which *Aurum* is indicated. Enchainment of the soul to the material world is always associated with premature aging of the physical body. The "hardness" that has been practiced outwardly also acts internally, leading to early sclerosis. This affects primarily heart and circulation, but other organs can be sympathetically affected—the liver for example (cirrhosis).[7]

Diseases for which Gold Is Indicated as a Remedy

The first warning signal is usually hypertension, frequently coupled with redness of the face and a slightly swollen appearance. If patients ignore this warning and do not change their life, a heart attack may occur under particular stress. Alternatively, such patients may be confronted with life crises that make no apparent sense but cause their entire value system to collapse. Marriage falls apart through death or separation; their children get into trouble, perhaps falling into a drug scene; everything goes wrong in business and irrecoverable losses mount. It is not surprising that under such changed circumstances the values, the meaning, the very foundations that sustained one's life seem to be gone. But what is specifically characteristic of this type is that their mode of dynamic activity implodes and gives way to dull, apathetic brooding. Practically overnight, individuals who were once full of energy fall into depression and melancholia. Depending on the patient's constitution, such cases may also be subject to heart attack. Yet no matter how the disease expresses itself, the affected

---

7   This characterization of the *Aurum* patient is based on various homeopathic descriptions published in *Documenta Homoeopathica*, vol. 1 and 4, Haug Verlag, Heidelberg, 1981.

organ, the site of the pathology, is always really the heart, even in cases of depression.

When such "success persons" lie incapacitated in bed, the first dutiful visitors tend to be employees and, later, friends. However, if they remain unwell for long, visitors become fewer and fewer; no one really knows what to talk about with them. Patients are seized by unbearable restlessness, impatience, and disappointment. They are enraged by a "failed" medical establishment. They blame the whole world and finally turn on themselves, as well, with self-reproaches and guilt. Never will they be able to get over the misfortune; everything that follows will be dark and desolate without the tiniest ray of light. Now they need the gold process as a remedy.

Why the gold process? The "success person" is dominated by the will; the soul life is directed completely outward, toward affecting the surrounding world. The inherent danger of this orientation is that, over time, they gradually lose inner harmony. The necessary correspondence between inner development and outer life is not guided and formed by the "I"; instead they are ruled by a peculiar dynamic that can be described as arbitrary. Because the demands and behavior of such individuals are immoderate, they lose their human center. Thus when failures and blows of fate come, they catch these people off guard and throw them all the more off course.

The Gold Process and Human Development

The gold process is the "process of the center" because it unites center and periphery. The periphery is perceived and gathered together in the heart, and from the heart a stream goes out again affecting the periphery. This dynamic can be symbolically portrayed as a circle with a point in the middle, the sign for the Sun and the gold process.

When the stage of consciousness known as the consciousness soul has been developed, it enables human beings to experience both perspectives—that of the center and that of the periphery.

Only now can they become truly aware how they affect the world around them. Only now can they objectively judge their own actions from the periphery. Only now can they develop moral judgment and true awareness of individual responsibility. Moreover, as individuals, they now experience themselves as entirely on their own, as individuals, and so are able to recognize themselves in their individuality. In this process, they also gain an objective distance from themselves.

With this new consciousness, questions may arise in the soul about one's hidden motivations. Why did I react in a certain way within a particular situation? The background to these questions now arises from the soul's depths, and it may reveal that our behavior has not been simply a "perfectly justified response" to outer circumstances, but was dominated by our own needs, longings, and wishes. What we previously saw as a reasonable reaction we now see as motivated by egoism. We were convinced that we were sacrificing ourselves for the sake of others; now we discover that we were motivated essentially by a need for recognition and self-affirmation. The "consciousness-soul attitude" makes it possible for us to look objectively at our inner world in all its nuances. Under these conditions a genuine sense of moral responsibility can develop.

Until the consciousness soul has developed, a human being lives entirely in the soul configuration called the "sentient and intellectual soul." One of its characteristics is that such individuals experience themselves as centers of activity and the surrounding world as their backdrop. At this self-centered stage of soul life, true self-knowledge is impossible. Sensations and feelings revolve directly around one's own person; world issues are one-sidedly related to oneself and are therefore experienced in a linear and causal way. It may be added that we are now living in a time of great transition, when the development of new soul faculties coincides with the effects of rampant technological expansion, so that the demands placed on the human being have reached a peak. At such pivotal periods in world history, an untrained consciousness and deficient self-knowledge may have devastating consequences.

People in the phase of the sentient and intellectual soul who tend toward a pyknic body type and a choleric temperament are oriented to a special degree toward the world around themselves, and if the *Aurum* process is disturbed in them they very easily lose inner equilibrium. Since they are in their active phase, such people are rarely ill, which enables them to accomplish so much. However, because they experience themselves as centers of the world and relate everything back to themselves, their actions are motivated primarily by egoism. As discussed, their outward success gives them the opportunity to enjoy the comfortable side of life fully, which binds them to materialism. The path of spiritualizing the inner life—recognizing the spiritual nature of the human individuality—is unavailable to them. Thus the breakthrough of the consciousness soul is delayed, and when it finally does occur, it is all the more powerful. With this breakthrough the old values, such as security and satisfaction based on possessions, become questionable—indeed, senseless. This great shift occurs dramatically and is frequently accompanied by serious illness.

The soul dynamic of the "will person" is best illustrated by the phenomenon of light. Light is not experienced until it strikes the surface of an object. It makes the object visible, and through the appearance of surfaces of objects turned toward the light we experience space. In the empty space between the objects, the light remains imperceptible, although only here is it actually present in its true nature. We are accustomed to take the perception of illuminated surfaces for the experience of light itself. The brighter the surface appears, the more light we believe we are experiencing; we identify the flood of light reflected by objects with light itself.

Will people experience their soul in a similar way. When they exert their soul-spiritual force, they experience it only in the world around them, on the "surfaces" that this force encounters. Nonetheless, they believe they are experiencing their true being. Given the dynamic of their soul life, it is impossible for such people to recognize that this force lives in an essentially spiritual realm—an intermediate space void of matter—and that it requires development. Thus when tragic events transpire, and when the "surfaces" fall apart—the surfaces through which they were accustomed to experiencing their selfhood, or "light," they believe that this, too, has "gone out." It is no longer possible for will individuals to experience their own soul light through the surrounding world and the soul itself experiences inner darkness. The link between themselves and others—between themselves as center points and those around them as periphery—falls apart.

The organic basis for maintaining this connection—primarily the heart and circulation—are the most affected in this process, but the soul life is always affected as well. When the link breaks, the heart may be affected with stenosis or infarction. At the same time, the heart is also involved in depression (however, to explain the details of this connection is beyond the scope of this work).

The Gold Process as the Way to the Heart

For this reason the gold process, as the keeper of balance between center and periphery, between spiritual individuality and material world (including our physical nature), is also the remedy for people in this predicament. Focused *Aurum* therapy that effectively supports the patient's gold process strives to release the "I" and astral body from bondage to the body and from the self-centered soul dynamic associated with it. Thus neutralized, self-centeredness can develop into selflessness; dominance into tolerance; existential anxiety into trust; and compulsive self-affirmation into genuine confidence. It is the step from sentient and intellectual soul to consciousness soul. A spiritual force develops that tests surface experiences for their spiritual validity. The spiritual principle of patients, the "I," now no longer only sees itself reflected in the surrounding world but able to occupy directly the perspective of the periphery. In this way, patients develop not only power of moral judgment and a sense of responsibility, but also new awareness of the true value of their own self. The health-bringing gold process helps extroverted will-persons to walk the path of soul purification toward spiritual inwardness. This is the Sun path depicted in the tale of "Hans in Luck."

Thus, Hans's example teaches *Aurum* patients to free themselves from fixation on external possessions, on material gold; they must learn to cease placing demands on life and accept events as dispensations, seeing the positive side even in blows of fate. Finding oneself and gaining a light heart—the counterparts of being success-driven and suffering cardiac stenosis or even a heart attack—are possible only by way of renunciation, outer loss, and mindfulness of the divine and spirit in one's own soul. The first, often laborious steps on this path must be taken by patients themselves, although in many cases they are possible only with the help of an empathetic physician. The last step, which truly frees and redeems the heart, often occurs suddenly and unexpectedly of its own accord. This is shown in the tale through the chance sinking of the stones in the well. Thus the fairy tale of "Hans in Luck" can be understood as a portrayal of the path of inner schooling that the *Aurum* patient needs to tread for personal healing. The remedy *Aurum* can be an aid on this path, but it cannot replace the readiness to travel it.

And so it turns out that what at first seemed paradoxical in this tale is actually the revelation of a deep and wisdom-filled truth.

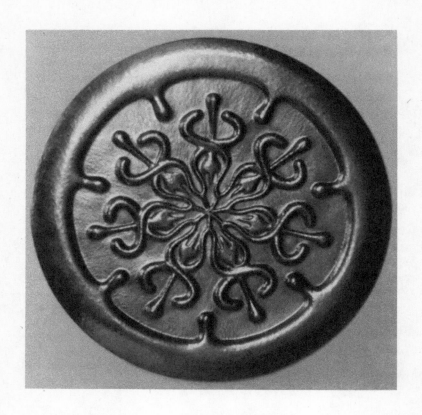

Mercury Seal

Copper as a Remedy: "Snow White"

Once upon a time in the middle of winter, when snowflakes were falling like feathers from Heaven, a queen sat at a window sewing, and the frame of the window was made of black ebony. And while she was sewing and looking out of the window at the snow, she pricked her finger with the needle, and three drops of blood fell upon the snow. And the red looked pretty upon the white snow, and she thought to herself, "Would that I had a child as white as snow, as red as blood, and as black as the wood of the window frame."

Soon after that she had a little daughter, who was as white as snow, and as red as blood, and her hair was as black as ebony; and she was therefore called Little Snow White. And when the child was born, the Queen died.

After a year had passed, the King took to himself another wife. She was a beautiful woman, but proud and haughty, and she could not bear that anyone else should surpass her in beauty. She had a wonderful mirror, and she stood in front of it and looked at herself in it and said, "Mirror, Mirror, on the wall, who in this land is the fairest of all?"

The mirror answered, "O Queen, you are the fairest of all!"

Then she was satisfied, for she knew that the mirror spoke the truth. But Snow White was growing up and grew more and more beautiful; and when she was seven years old she was as beautiful as the day, and more beautiful than the Queen herself. And once when the Quen asked her mirror, "Mirror, Mirror, on the wall, who in this land is the fairest of all?" it answered, "You are the fairest of all I see, but Snow White is a thousand times fairer than you."

Then the Queen was shocked and turned yellow and green with envy. From that hour, whenever she looked at Snow White, her heart heaved in her breast, she hated the girl so much. Envy and pride grew higher and higher in her heart like a weed, so that she had no peace day or night. She called a hunter and said, "Take the child away into the forest; I will no longer have her in my sight. Kill her, and bring me back her lungs and liver as a token." The hunter obeyed and took her away, but when he had drawn his knife and was about to pierce Snow White's innocent heart, she began to weep and said, "Ah, dear hunter, leave me my life! I will run away into the wild forest and never come home again."

She was so beautiful that the hunter took pity on her and said, "Run away, then, you poor child." *The wild beasts will soon have devoured you,* he thought, yet it seemed as if a stone had been rolled from his heart, since he no longer felt a need to kill her. And as a young boar just then came running by he stabbed it and cut out its lungs and liver and took them to the Queen as proof that the child was dead. The cook had to salt this, and the wicked Queen ate it and thought she had eaten Snow White's lungs and liver.

But now the poor child was all alone in the great forest, and so terrified that she looked at every leaf of every tree and did not know what to do. Then she began to run, and ran over sharp stones and through thorns, and the wild beasts ran past her, but did her no harm.

She ran as long as her feet would go until it was almost evening; then she saw a little cottage and went into it to rest herself. Everything in the cottage was small, but neater and cleaner than can be told. There was a table on which was a white cover, and seven little plates, and on each plate a little spoon; moreover, there were seven little knives and forks and seven little mugs. Against the wall stood seven little beds side by side and covered with Snow White counterpanes.

Little Snow White was so hungry and thirsty that she ate some vegetables and bread from each plate and drank a drop of wine from each mug, for she did not wish to take all from one only. Then, she was so tired she laid herself down on one of the little beds, but none of them suited her; one was too long, another too short, but at last she found that the seventh one was right, and so she remained in it, said a prayer, and went to sleep.

When it was quite dark the owners of the cottage came back; they were seven dwarfs who dug and delved in the mountains for ore. They lit their seven candles, and as it was not light within the cottage they saw that someone had been there, for everything was not in the same order in which they had left it.

The first said, "Who has been sitting on my chair?"

The second, "Who has been eating off my plate?"

The third, "Who has been taking some of my bread?"

The fourth, "Who has been eating my vegetables?"

The fifth, "Who has been using my fork?"

The sixth, "Who has been cutting with my knife?"

The seventh, "Who has been drinking out of my mug?"

Then the first looked round and saw that there was a little hole on his bed; he said, "Who has been getting into my bed?" The others came up and each called out, "Somebody has been lying in my bed, too." But the seventh, when he looked at his bed saw little Snow White lying asleep therein, he called the others, who came running up. They cried out with astonishment and brought their seven little candles, letting the light fall on little Snow White. "Oh, heavens! Oh, heavens!" they cried, "What a lovely child!" They were so glad that they did not wake her up but let her sleep on in the bed. And the seventh dwarf slept with his companions, one hour with each, and so got through the night.

When it was morning little Snow White awoke and was frightened when she saw the seven dwarfs. But they were friendly and asked her what her name was. "My name is Snow White," she answered.

"How have you come to our house?" said the dwarfs. Then she told them that her step-mother had wished to have her killed, but that the hunter had spared her life, and that she had run for the whole day until at last she had found their dwelling.

The dwarfs said, "If you will take care of our house, cook, make the beds, wash, sew and knit, and if you will keep everything neat and clean, you can stay with us and you shall want for nothing."

"Yes," said Snow White, "with all my heart," and she stayed with them. She kept the house for them; in the mornings they went to the mountains and looked for copper and gold; in the evenings they returned, and then their supper had to be ready. The girl was alone the whole day, so the good dwarfs warned her and said, "Beware of your step-mother, she will soon know that you are here; be sure to let no one come in."

But the Queen, believing that she had eaten Snow White's heart, could not but think that she was again the first and most beautiful of all; and she went to her mirror and said, "Mirror, Mirror, on the wall, who in this land is the fairest of all?"

And the glass answered, "You, O Queen, are fairest of all I see, but over the hills where the seven dwarfs dwell, Snow White is still alive and well, and she is a thousand times fairer than you." Then she was astounded, for she knew that the mirror never spoke falsely, and she knew that the hunter had betrayed her, and that little Snow White was still alive.

And so she thought and thought again how she might kill her, for so long as she was not the fairest in the whole land, envy let her have no rest. And when she had at last thought of something to do, she painted her face and dressed herself like an old peddler-woman, and no one could have known her. In this disguise she went over the seven mountains to the seven dwarfs and knocked at the door and cried, "Pretty things to sell, very cheap, very cheap."

Little Snow White looked out of the window and called out, "Good-day, my good woman; what have you to sell?"

"Good things, pretty things," she answered, "stay-laces of all colors." She pulled out one that was woven of brightly colored silk.

"I may let the worthy old woman in," thought Snow White, and she unbolted the door and bought the pretty laces. "Child," said the old woman, "what a fright you look; come, I will lace you properly for once." Snow White had no suspicion, but stood before her and let herself be laced with the new laces. But the old woman laced so quickly and laced so tightly that Snow White lost her breath and fell down as if dead. "Now I am the most beautiful," said the Queen to herself and ran away.

Not long after, in the evening, the seven dwarfs came home, but they were shocked when they saw their dear little Snow White lying on the ground, and that she neither stirred nor moved and seemed to be dead. They lifted her and, as they saw that she was laced too tightly, cut the laces. Then she began to breathe a little and after a while returned to life. When the dwarfs heard what had happened they said, "The old peddler-woman was no one else than the wicked Queen; take care and let no one come in when we are not with you."

But the wicked woman when she had reached home went in front of the glass and asked, "Mirror, Mirror, on the wall, who in this land is the fairest of all?"

And it answered as before, "You, O Queen, are fairest of all I see, but over the hills where the seven dwarfs dwell, Snow White is still alive and well, and she is a thousand times fairer than you. When she heard that, all her blood rushed to her heart with fear, for she saw plainly that little Snow White was again alive. "But now," she said, "I will think of something that shall put an end to you," and by the help of witchcraft, which she understood, she made a poisonous comb. Then she disguised herself and took the shape of another old woman.

So she went over the seven mountains to the seven dwarfs, knocked at the door, and cried, "Good things to sell cheap, cheap!"

Little Show-white looked out and said, "Go away; I cannot let anyone come in."

"I suppose you can look," said the old woman, and pulled the poisonous comb out and held it up. It pleased the girl so well that she let herself be beguiled and opened the door. When they had made a bargain the old woman said, "Now I will comb you properly for once."

Poor little Snow White had no suspicion and let the old woman do as she pleased, but hardly had she put the comb in her hair than the poison in it took effect, and the girl fell senseless. "You paragon of beauty," said the wicked woman, "you are done for now," and she went away.

Fortunately, it was almost evening, when the seven dwarfs would come home. When they saw Snow White lying as if dead upon the ground, they at once suspected the step-mother, and they looked and found the poisoned comb. Scarcely had they taken it out when Snow White came to herself and told them what had happened. Then they warned her once more to be upon her guard and to open the door to no one.

The Queen, at home, went before the glass and said, "Mirror, Mirror, on the wall, who in this land is the fairest of all?"

Then it answered as before, "You, O Queen, are fairest of all I see, but over the hills where the seven dwarfs dwell, Snow White is still alive and well, and she is a thousand times fairer than you.

When she heard the glass speak thus she trembled and shook with rage. "Snow White shall die," she cried, "even if it costs me my life!" With this, she went into a quite secret, lonely room where no one ever came, and there she made a poisonous apple. Outside it looked pretty, white with a red cheek, so that every one who saw it longed for it; but whoever ate a piece of it must surely die.

When the apple was ready, she painted her face, and dressed herself up as a country woman. And so she went over the seven mountains to the seven dwarfs. She knocked at the door. Show White put her head out of the window and said, "I cannot let anyone in; the seven dwarfs have forbidden me."

"It is all the same to me," answered the woman, "I shall soon get rid of my apples. There, I will give you one."

"No," said Snow White, "I dare not take anything."

"Are you afraid of poison?" said the old woman. "Look, I will cut the apple in two pieces; you eat the red cheek, and I will eat the white." The apple was so cunningly made that only the red cheek was poisoned. Show-white longed for the fine apple, and when she saw that the woman ate part of it she could resist no longer and stretched out her hand and took the poisonous half. But hardly had she a bite of it in her mouth than she fell dead. Then the Queen looked at her with a dreadful look and laughed aloud and said, "White as snow, red as blood, black as ebony wood! This time the dwarfs cannot wake you up again."

And when she asked of the Mirror at home, "Mirror, Mirror, on the wall, who in this land is the fairest of all?" it answered at last, "Oh, Queen, in this land you are fairest of all." Then her envious heart had peace, insofar as an envious heart can have peace.

The dwarfs, when they came home in the evening, found Snow White lying upon the ground. She no longer breathed and was dead. They lifted her, looked to see if they could find anything poisonous, unlaced her, combed her hair, washed her with water and wine, but it was all of no use; the poor child was dead and remained dead. They laid her upon a bier, and all seven of them sat round it and wept for her; they wept three days long.

Then they were going to bury her, but she still looked as if she were living and still had her pretty red cheeks. They said, "We could not bury her in the dark ground," and they had a transparent coffin of glass made so that she could be seen from all sides. They laid her in it and wrote her name upon it in golden letters and that she was a king's daughter. Then they put the coffin out upon the mountain, and one of them always stayed by it and watched it. And birds came, too, and wept for Snow White, first an owl, then a raven, and last a dove.

Now Snow White lay a very long time in the coffin, and she did not change but looked as if she were asleep, for she was as white as snow, as red as blood, and her hair was as black as ebony.

It happened, however, that a king's son came into the forest and went to the dwarfs' house to spend the night. He saw the coffin on the mountain and the beautiful Snow White within it and read what was written upon it in golden letters. Then he said to the dwarfs, "Let me have the coffin; I will give you whatever you want for it."

But the dwarfs answered, "We will not part with it for all the gold in the world."

Then he said, "Let me have it as a gift, for I cannot live without seeing Snow White. I will honor and prize her as my dearest possession." As he spoke in this way the good dwarfs took pity on him and gave him the coffin.

Now the King's son had it carried away by his servants on their shoulders, and it happened that they stumbled over a tree-stump, and with the shock the poisonous piece of apple which Snow White had bitten off came out of her throat. Before long, she opened her eyes, lifted the lid of the coffin, sat up, and was once more alive. "Oh, heavens, where am I?" she cried.

The King's son, full of joy, said, "You are with me," and told her what had happened. He said, "I love you more than everything in the world; come with me to my father's palace, and you shall be my wife." Snow White was willing, went with him, and their wedding was held with great show and splendor.

But Snow White's wicked step-mother was also invited to the feast. When she had arrayed herself in beautiful clothes, she went before the Mirror and said, "Mirror, Mirror, on the wall, who in this land is the fairest of all?" The glass answered, "You, O Queen, are fairest of all I see, but the young queen is a thousand times fairer than you."

Then the wicked woman uttered a curse and was so wretched, so utterly wretched, that she knew not what to do. At first she would not go to the wedding at all, but she had no peace and must go to see the young Queen. When she went in, she knew Snow White; she stood still with rage and fear and could not stir. But iron slippers had already been put upon the fire, and they were brought in with tongs and set before her. Then she was forced to put on the red-hot shoes and dance until she dropped dead. But over the hills where the seven dwarfs dwell, "Snow White is still alive and well and a thousand times fairer than you."[1]

~

Following the gold process, we come to the copper process, and as a source of insight we turn to "Snow White." Since ancient times copper has been associated with the planet Venus and with the goddess of love and beauty who bears the same name. Thus in describing the copper process we are at the same time describing essential qualities of the Venus sphere.

When the "I" passes into the Venus sphere on its incarnation path, it enters the realm of the "subsolar" planets. These latter are paired with specific "suprasolar" planets, which have (in part) opposite characteristics, and in this way the Venus sphere is paired with the Mars sphere. We shall go into more detail on this aspect below, but it bears noting here that this opposition is also reflected in the corresponding fairy tales. Thus, Snow White has her exact opposite in Iron Hans, and as we examine "Snow White" it will be useful to bear in mind its contrasts with "Iron Hans." As before, however, we will consider the metal itself before going into the fairy tale.

The Metal Copper

The copper minerals are remarkable for their luminosity and variety of coloration. In copper ores we meet with blues, greens, reds, and even purples. Malachite, azurite, and dioptase[2] all seem to be competing for the prize in color splendor and charm. No other metal transforms itself into so many and such various forms as copper.

The gamut of colors displayed by the copper ores is connected with their water content; they seem to "hoard" water in an organized

---

1   The Harvard Classics, 1909–14; http://www.bartleby.com/17/2/25.html (revised).

2   *Dioptase* is an emerald-green to bluish-green, transparent to translucent copper cyclosilicate mineral.

form. Magnificent blue (copper sulfate) and green (copper chloride) crystals are formed by soluble copper salts, which contain up to 35% water. When the water is evaporated by heating, not only the color but also the crystal form disappears. These phenomena observable in copper—colorfulness, mutability, and combining ability—also point toward the therapeutic qualities of the metal and its compounds, which we will discuss in more detail.

At one time mirrors were commonly made from sheets of polished copper. Such mirrors were reddish and gave the reflected face a lovely rosy tint. The mirror of Aphrodite, the goddess's traditional symbol, is also pictured as copper.[3]

The Mood of the Tale

"Snow White" is surely one of the best known in the Grimms' collection. It is easy to identify with the heroine and empathize with her sufferings. Her story touches the heart; her innocence, her helplessness and her weakness arouse whole-hearted sympathy. The account of her housekeeping for the dwarves, tidying and cooking, appeals to the imagination. And watching Snow White succumb again and again to the seductive arts of her evil stepmother draws her close to us on a human level. While the king's son in "Iron Hans" takes the initiative and acts with sureness, it is the opposite with Snow White; hers is a loving and devoted but rather passive nature that submits and suffers. Everything in this tale is permeated with innocence, tenderness and beauty, speaking to the depths of the soul. We are reminded of the words Rudolf Steiner used to characterize the Venus sphere; it is the source of the forces that endow human beings with a soulful sensibility.[4] It is entirely a sphere of "reverie," transforming everything into dream

---

3   As late as the Middle Ages, Aphrodite was frequently shown with her traditional symbol, a mirror; see Albertus Magnus, *The Book of Secrets of the Virtues of Herbs, Stones, and Certain Beasts* (from *Naturalia Alberti Magni*, 1548), Oxford, 1973.

4   Steiner, *Eurythmy as Visible Speech*, Dornach, July 7, 1924.

images.[5] This quality of the Venus sphere is reflected in the mood of the fairy tale.

The Main Motifs of the Tale

First let us look at the motifs that set the mood of this tale and compare them with those of "Iron Hans." Toward the end of "Iron Hans," we encountered the motif of three successive colors, red–white–black. These appear in the armor of the knight who thrice wins the golden apple for his accomplishments—that is, for his past development. In "Snow White," on the other hand, the motif of the three colors is already present from the start, when the queen wishes for a child as white as snow, as red as blood, and as black as ebony. So here the three colors express a beginning, not a culmination as in "Iron Hans." And the different order, white–red–black, prefigures a path of purification. This is embodied in the child who fulfills the queen's wishes and so is named Snow White.

It is not accidental that the sequence of colors is different in the two tales. In "Snow White," the color triad is introduced with the image of white snowflakes, highlighting a characteristic motif of the tale. Steiner indicates that snow crystals, with their six-pointed-star principle, help us understand the forces that are actually at work in matter.[6] By contemplating the white snow cover we can recognize what fills the world with materiality; we can experience the "weaving and being" of matter in the world. This is what Hermann Beckh, too, perceives in the ice crystals of snowflakes; it is as if in them the starry veil of the goddess Isis-Venus becomes a material veil.[7] And the image of the drops of blood falling from the finger of the expecting mother and mixing with the snow (a motif not unique to this tale)

---

5   Steiner, *Initiationswissenschaft und Sternenerkenntnis,* Dornach, July 27, 1923.

6   Steiner, *Spiritual Beings in the Heavenly Bodies and the Kingdoms of Nature,* Helsinki, Apr. 3, 1912.

7   Beckh, *Alchymie. Vom Geheimnis der Stoffeswelt* (Alchemy: Secrets of the World of Substance).

speaks of the union of a spiritual individuality with the mysterious forces of the material world. When the human "I" unites with the world of matter, death comes into being, which is signified here by the final color in the triad, black. Thus when the polarity of white and red becomes the triad of white, red, and black, a static opposition is transformed into a dynamic process.

Significantly, the longing for a child, for the incarnation of a new being, is alluded to in certain fairy tales through the three colors white, red and black. In another sense as well the mystery of earthly incarnation can be discovered in the three colors; their physiological interaction in the organism produces the color of "peach blossom," or "incarnadine," the healthy flesh tone of white-skinned humanity. A lecture by Steiner sheds interesting light on this point: "Just as I have

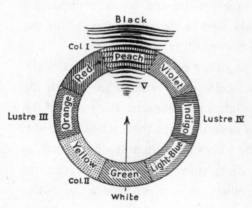

just let yellow and blue radiate in from the left and right, now let this wavy part, where black and white are constantly playing in, be shone through, irradiated by red.... If I had been able to find the right shade, then by letting red shine into these interpenetrating waves of black and white, I would get peach-blossom."[8]

In producing a healthy flesh color, the functions of the renal system play a critical role, as an exhaustive study by Heinz H. Schöffler has demonstrated.[9] Disease tendencies or actual diseases of the kidneys are frequently apparent to the attentive observer from the patient's complexion. We will return to the significance of copper in the renal system when we come to the disease pictures.

8   Steiner, *Color*, Dornach, May 6 and 7, 1921.

9   H. H. Schöffler, "Niere und Nebenniere" [Kidney and Adrenal Gland]. *Beiträge zu einer Erweiterung der Heilkunst*, Stuttgart, Apr. 1975.

Let us now explore further motifs of the fairy tale. The plot of the story hinges on a stepmother who cannot tolerate being outshone in beauty and therefore wishes to kill her surpassingly radiant stepdaughter. Beauty and vanity are thus two motifs of the tale. The stepmother possesses a wonderful mirror—one of copper, we may assume—that always tells the truth. As long as it can assure her that she is the "fairest in the land," she is content. But when Snow White reaches the age of seven, the mirror suddenly speaks of her as "a thousand times fairer." The reference to the age of seven is a clear indication that the fairy tale is alluding not to external beauty, but to something within.

The mirror is a many-layered motif. Numerous mythological images depict Venus with the traditional symbol of the mirror in her hand. This is significant in connection with the copper process, for beauty cannot be directly experienced. To experience oneself as beautiful one needs an external reflection. In other words one must become self-absorbed like the stepmother. Below it will become clear that this is an imaginative insight into a particular aspect of the copper process.

The motif of reflection in this tale addresses yet another and deeper level of our existence. According to widespread mythological traditions, matter had its origin when certain divine beings fell in love with their own image reflected in the primeval waters, and descended to unite themselves with it.[10] "Snow White" seems to contain an intimation of these mysteries, as it speaks of the soul's progressive descent into matter through a series of phases culminating in Snow White's entombment in a glass coffin, where she has entered a crystalline state as it were. Thus from the copper perspective this tale depicts the incarnation path of the "I" into bodily nature and the dangers that this entails.

Returning to the plot of the tale, we now find Snow White fleeing her murderous stepmother. Far across the seven mountains she finds

---

10   Jung, "Erlösungsvorstellungen in der Alchemie" [Redemption Ideas in Alchemy] (Walter Verlag Olten, 1985), p. 78.

refuge at the home of the seven dwarves. Three times the stepmother, disguised as a countrywoman going about her work in the daytime, succeeds in approaching Snow White and doing her harm. The first two times, when the dwarves come home they are able to bring her back to life by night. The third time, however, the stepmother has succeeded in poisoning Snow White so severely that the dwarves can no longer save her. In deep mourning they lay the seemingly dead princess in a glass coffin, over which they keep careful watch.

This dramatic episode offers a description of the functional and physiological action of the copper process in the organism. During the nighttime the action of the copper process is anabolic: building up, nourishing and regenerating. During the daytime, with the intense incursion of the forces of consciousness, it acts catabolically, breaking down bodily substance. This can reach the point where it produces cramps. In conditions of cramping, consciousness becomes so dominant that it appears at places where it is normally not present; and this is experienced as pain.

The stepmother represents the effects of daytime consciousness, when the copper process acts toxically. The kind of toxic conditions suffered by Snow White can be recognized as disease pictures in which the copper process is disturbed and its unwholesome effects cannot be absorbed. The seven dwarves, who come home in the evening to find Snow White unconscious and twice succeed in saving her, can be seen as an imagination of the manifold positive activities of the copper process during the night, when it acts regeneratively and is able to counteract the poisoning. Further on we will look more closely at these disease pictures and also examine the third picture, when Snow White lies in the glass coffin.

Another essential difference between Snow White and the king's son in "Iron Hans" is the way they approach their fates. After acquiring his golden hair more or less innocently, the king's son becomes master of his fate. From now on he sets his own course in life; the impulses always come from him. How different Snow White;

everything that happens in her life happens *to her*. She is unable to withstand the temptations that meet her. In short, she is not master but victim of her fate. Yet this does not mean that she is helpless, for at every critical juncture other powers come to her aid. Although Snow White fails to see through the tests devised by her stepmother and must suffer the consequences, her very failure opens up the possibility of purification, of overcoming her weaknesses. And so it is that Snow White's story, too, can come to a happy end.

Thus the chief characters in "Snow White" and "Iron Hans" develop in diametrically opposed directions; like Venus and Mars, their corresponding divinities, they stand in polar opposition.

The Polarization of the Copper Process

Now we can enter into the details of the plot. When the mirror answers for the first time that Snow White is the fairest in all the land, the child has just reached the age of seven. How is this to be understood? Around the seventh year of life every human being undergoes a crucial change. The ether body (or life-body) is released from the close connection to the body that it has held until this stage of childhood, which allows some of the freed formative forces to metamorphose into the capacity for thinking. At this point the child has reached readiness for school. From a purely external point of view, this change is signaled by the appearance of the permanent teeth.

The copper sphere plays an important role in this transformation.[11] Up to this point its activity in the organism was wholly a formative metabolic function. Now it is partially released from this and enters increasingly into the soul life. Imagination and memory develop—powers which depend on the copper process. And it is largely thanks to the copper process that the soul is able to develop a sense for what is beautiful and admirable. This gives children of this age the particular radiance that we experience as their charm. And

---

11   Walter Holtzapfel, "Der Kupferprozeß in der kindlichen Entwicklung" [The Copper Process in Child Development], *Beiträge zu einer Erweiterung der Heilkunst"* 5/6, 1955, Stuttgart.

this is the transformation that has now taken place in Snow White; the copper process has manifested in her as a soul faculty, openness to the world and the power of devotion. She represents the liberated copper forces of the soul; she is now truly the fairest in all the land.

As mentioned before, the stepmother, too, personifies the copper process, only its earthly, self-centered form. In her case, beauty can be experienced only in external reflection—that is, in vanity. Thus the stepmother and Snow White are personifications of closely related yet antithetical aspects of the copper sphere that can both become active in every human being. The polarization of the two streams begins the moment when the being of Copper becomes free in the soul realm. This is why the stepmother now rejects Snow White. In fact, she goes so far as to order a hunter to kill her and bring her the lungs and liver as proof, intending to have them cooked in salt and consume them. These two organs have a direct relationship to the polar copper processes, while the kidneys are associated with the unified copper process. The lungs, the organ through which we open ourselves to the environment, stand for the openness and devotion aspect of copper. They mediate the continuous breath stream that connects the human being with the environment. Each of us inhales air that others have exhaled; in this realm there is no separation. The oxygen that is taken in with the air makes possible a kind of internal combustion, hence it may fairly be said that with the air we receive fire. This fire-air makes possible an inner purification, which (according to Steiner) can lead the being of man to higher spheres.[12] The liver, in contrast, is the seat of self-centeredness, the egoistic principle proper. Steiner speaks of the liver as the organ that "stuffs everything egoistic into the human being." From this point of view the liver must be connected with the self-centered copper process of "vanity."

Steiner elaborates further that between the liver system (including gallbladder and spleen) and the lung system, there stands the activity

---

12   Steiner, *The Influence of Spiritual Beings on Man*, Berlin, Jan. 6, 1908.

of the kidneys.[13] These have a harmonizing action, balancing out irregular activity in one or the other of the mentioned organ systems. In this way they prevent "encroachments" in these vital functional realms of the organism.

Copper and the Seven Life Processes

Rudolf Steiner speaks of seven life processes or anabolic functions of the organism, which are breathing, warming, nourishing, secreting, maintaining, growing, and reproducing.[14] Let us review the well-known images of this tale in their relation to copper.

The hunter, feeling pity for Snow White, does not kill her but lets her go. In her place he kills a boar and brings its lungs and liver to the queen. Snow White wanders through the forest and eventually finds refuge with the seven dwarves over the seven mountains. "Mountains," as Pernety explains, is an alchemical symbol for "metals," the foundational forces of the world.[15] The daily task of the dwarves, after all, is to "dig and delve" for ore in the mountains.

No one is home when Snow White enters the dwarves' house, but she finds a table set for seven. From each plate Snow White takes a small amount of food, from each glass she drinks a drop of wine, and in this way she satisfies her hunger and thirst. Then she tries out the seven little beds, lies down in the one that best fits her, and goes to sleep. When it is dark the seven dwarves come home and find Snow White asleep. How are we to interpret these images? The seven dwarves, as representatives of the metal forces in their sevenfold ordering, can be connected with the seven life processes mentioned above; for in "Snow White" these seven life processes appear under their particular copper aspect, which has a special relationship to the warming, nourishing, anabolic

13 Steiner, *An Occult Physiology*, Prague, Mar. 23, 1911.

14 Bauer, Dunat, and Golowin, *Lexikon der Symbole*.

15 Steiner, *The Riddle of Man*, Dornach, Aug. 12, 1916.

functions of the life processes. This is shown in the image of Snow White eating and drinking from the meal table of the seven dwarves, which implies that each dwarf represents one of the seven anabolic life processes. Their questions, repeated seven times in variation, point to aspects of the seven life processes by use of telling images: "Who has been sitting on my chair?"; "Who has been eating off my plate?"; "Who has been taking some of my bread?"; "Who has been eating my vegetables?"; "Who has been using my fork?"; "Who has been cutting with my knife?"; and "Who has been drinking out of my mug?"

We have seen that the copper process, once it has become free in the soul realm, acts catabolically on the life processes. While it was intimately bound to them, it had formed a kind of sheath for them until around the seventh year of life. Now this protective covering is largely removed, for when the copper process is liberated in the soul realm there is also a change in its functions, which until then were anabolic. When it begins to act on the consciousness level, its action is catabolic. This is indicated in the questions of the seven dwarves. Copper has a special relation to one of the seven life processes in particular: that of nourishing. This suggests to us that the bed that Snow White sleeps in is that of the dwarf who represents this process, because it fits her exactly.

The Copper Process in the Soul Realm

The next morning, Snow White tells the dwarves her story—why she had to run away from home and how she found their house. They allow her to remain with them, but in return she must "take care of [their] house." In other words, the soul must make and keep order within itself. The copper process generates longing in the soul, exposing it to temptations that bring it into "disorder." What Snow White must learn is to resist these weaknesses. Most significantly, the dwarves warn Snow White against her stepmother—that is, against the vain and self-centered impulses of her soul. In spite of her good intentions Snow White succumbs to immature desires because she does not recognize their danger; what she sees is an honest peddler, not her stepmother in disguise. As a result, when the dwarves return from work in the evening they find her laced up so tight that she is unable to breathe and is lying unconscious on the ground. The condition into which Snow White is put by the laces can be interpreted as the first disease picture connected with the copper process. No longer mastered by the "I"-organization, the copper process slips out of control and causes congestion, to which in turn the organism reacts with cramping. In their most striking form, spasmodic conditions connected with the copper process express themselves as asthma. The asthmatic is unable to exhale properly, so that stale air builds up in the lungs. Those asthma attacks that respond well to potentized *Cuprum metallicum* are precisely the kind in which the patient's chest feels constricted, as if bound in tight straps.[16]

It is not until night that the cramping, the build-up of air in the lungs (the "lacing"), can be released, since at night the anabolic process gain the upper hand over the catabolic processes. This process of release and integration can be effectively supported with copper as a remedy, particularly when used as long-term therapy.

Let us not ignore an apparent contradiction between our interpretation of the fairy tale and the remedy picture for asthma. In the remedy picture, the symptoms worsen at night. In particular, the asthma attacks that respond to *Cuprum* preparations commonly occur around three o'clock in the morning. Yet perhaps this makes sense when we consider that by this time the physiological daytime pattern is beginning. The liver resumes its metabolic activity at this time; and when its functions are disturbed, this has repercussions on the entire organism, aggravating the breathlessness.

---

16   Köhler, *Handbook of Homeopathy.*

The Copper Process in the Ether Body

There follow two more attacks by the stepmother, each of which can be understood as a disease picture based on a disturbed copper process. In the first of these, the stepmother makes a poisoned comb, disguises herself again and seeks out the dwarves' dwelling. Once again Snow White is beguiled and cannot resist trying on one of the pretty combs. When the evil old woman sticks the poisoned comb into her hair, Snow White falls senseless to the ground.

Let us examine this image. This time the attack relates to the hair. Hair is an expression of the etheric forces and is connected with the liver. It plays a significant role in a great many fairy tales—one need only think of "The Goose Girl," "Iron Hans," or "Rapunzel," and in each case it is an expression of something related to the etheric body. In the case of "Snow White," the insertion of a poisoned comb into the hair pictorially expresses congestion in the ether body. The chief organ of the ether body is the liver, and so the congestion concerns chiefly this organ. A disease picture that we must associate with this congestion is epilepsy. Epileptic fits are frequently triggered by congestion in the liver region that is suddenly released upward into the nerve-sense system, leading to tonic-clonic seizures.[17] And in epilepsy too, copper proves to be one of the most important remedies—therapeutic confirmation that epilepsy can be connected with a disturbed copper process.

In the story it is once again the seven dwarves—the anabolic life processes—that have the power to release the congestion. They find the poisoned comb in Snow White's hair, and the moment they pull it out she regains consciousness. Once again the nighttime anabolic processes are able to overcome the cramping.

The Copper Process in the Physical Body

Let us review the images of the third poisoning now. When the stepmother learns from her mirror that her second attack has failed

---

17   Steiner, *Education for Special Needs.*

she is seized by uncontrollable rage and immediately sets about devising a final deadly attack. Again she comes to Snow White in the guise of harmless country-woman, this time bearing an artfully poisoned apple. By now, Snow White ought to know better than to accept things from strangers, yet at the sight of the apple she is overcome by desire. The stepmother overcomes her last hesitancy by demonstratively eating one half (the half not poisoned) herself. Snow White takes the other half and bites into it. A single bite suffices and she falls down dead. When the dwarves come home at night and find Snow White in this condition, they cannot find its cause, and so no help is possible. They must accept that Snow White is dead. Yet because the lovely pinkness does not fade from her cheeks and she seems as fresh as a living person, they cannot put her in a grave but instead have a glass coffin fashioned in which Snow White can be viewed from all sides. In gold letters they write her name on it, and that she is a king's daughter. Then they place the coffin up on a mountain and take turns watching over it. All the animals of the forest come to mourn Snow White.

How are these images to be interpreted? The apple recalls the story of the Fall from the Bible, but unlike Eve, Snow White does not fully swallow the bite she has taken; it remains stuck in her throat. The image matches that of an externally manifesting goiter—that is, hypothyroidism with swelling of the thyroid gland. When we study this comparison more carefully, we discover that it is not merely a chance, external correspondence. Snow White in the glass coffin with the piece of poisoned apple in her throat is the soul-image of a person suffering from hypothyroidism. We shall go into this in greater detail.

The Disease Pictures and Dynamic of the Copper Process

Now let us survey the three disease pictures and attempt to understand the dynamic of the fairy tale in terms of the functional and physiological aspects of the human organism in which the copper process plays a critical role. A great range of motifs is united in

"Snow White," distributed among the different characters: longing for a child; envy, hunger for power and dominance; grace, beauty, and devotion; wisdom, loyalty, and nobility of character. But the most important motif is surely beauty—inner beauty. Snow White's beauty is so great that it touches the dwarves, representatives of the elemental kingdoms.

The physiological basis for the development of beauty as a soul quality is found chiefly in the kidneys; and they are the specific focus of the activity of the copper process. After substance has been "unlocked" and enlivened by the liver, it is ensouled in the kidneys and passes over into the domain of the individualized human soul. At the same time the kidneys are also the site of waste removal, of purification. Substances that cannot be "internalized," i.e., ensouled, are excreted. If this renal function is imbalanced, the result may be cramping. Asthma in particular may also result, because the renal system is closely connected with pulmonary activity (as we have already discussed). In the complex physiological process it is also possible that a disturbed kidney process can enter into a special relationship to the liver function, and this irregularity can lead to epileptic disorders. While the relationship to the lungs tends to play out on the soul level, the relationship to the liver manifests in the etheric.

The renal system, however, is by no means the only area in which the copper process is active in the organism. If it were limited in this way, our entire bodily substance would be at the mercy of the self-centered human ego with all its fantastical wishes and deceptive longings. Our bodily nature would be cut off from the cosmic-spiritual laws that formed and structured it. Hence the copper process possesses a further dynamic whose action is centered in the thyroid gland. Here it is raised to a higher level of existence. The thyroid gland draws the copper process completely into the physical body. Through warmth, this organ enables the inner "melting down" and re-forming that purifies the body. The thyroid regulates the basal metabolic rate, while toward the periphery it allows bodily substance to become hard and lifeless on its outer surface. In this way the thyroid makes our body as a whole into a "vessel" that is capable of receiving the intentions of a higher plane of existence. In other words, it is through the copper process that our bodily nature can be transformed to become the expression of higher spirituality. However, if this process escapes the full guidance of the "I," thyroid disease may result. In this connection we can see Snow White's glass coffin as the image of a human body that has become crystalline, a body in which the individual soul nature has been completely subdued and hardens.

Whereas irregular renal activity endangers the true self, or essence of the human being, by exposing us to deceptive desires and longings, a disturbed thyroid function threatens us with hardening tendencies. The thyroid gland has an important role not only in the regulation of metabolic activity but also in the maintenance and alteration of the form of the physical body. This function of the thyroid gland can be demonstrated quite impressively with frogs. In the frog, the metamorphosis from tadpole to frog—the step from aquatic to terrestrial life—is triggered by the thyroid hormone. When tadpoles are injected with this hormone, they shed their tails, transforming their fins into feet and their gills into lungs. Thus in frogs the thyroid hormone enables their maturity for life on Earth. When there is decreased thyroid functioning, this step cannot be taken to completion.

In the human being, the transformations leading to puberty and earthly maturity are also closely connected with thyroid activity. In the human being, however, this transformation goes deeper; it is more inward directed. When thyroid function is insufficient, the necessary changes cannot take place. The organism hardens outward toward the periphery in the attempt to preserve its earlier form. It wants to become a crystal that can maintain its form pure and unaltered— Snow White in her glass coffin. It wants to retain its purity and so resists a maturation process that would entail profound upheavals. On this point the contrast between Snow White and Iron Hans is particularly obvious. For the king's son the goal is always confrontation and change. He fights to win the golden apple, which is to say he is fighting for earthly maturity, which is his goal.

Copper is also a specific remedy for thyroid diseases of this type. Low thyroid function is treated with *Olivenit* D6 in conjunction with other preparations, while for high thyroid function *Cuprite* is the chief remedy.[18] These therapeutic links between copper compounds and thyroid diseases can offer us valuable support in our interpretive attempts.

The Shock that Awakens to New Life

It is beyond the power of the seven dwarves to save Snow White in her poisoned, rigidified state. This time it is a deeper poisoning than the healing life processes of the night can undo. Only a profound shock can release her from such rigidity. The fairy tale describes it in the following way: The king's son has received the coffin as a gift from the faithful dwarves, but the servants carrying it to his castle stumble on the way. Snow White receives such a jolt that the piece of apple is loosened from her throat and falls out. Freed of the poisoned morsel, she comes to life again. And as we see in the imagery of the fairy tale, the jolt has brought about not only healing, but also transformation: Snow White falls in love with the king's son and marries him. The wedding is celebrated "with great show and splendor."

When the soul has undergone maturation and transformation, the vain, egoistic copper process, as well as the associated congestion and cramping, is overcome. Hence at the wedding the evil stepmother, the embodiment of this negative aspect of the copper process, must dance in red-hot shoes until she drops dead. In dancing, we experience ourselves and the world as one. We are carried by the music

---

18   Steiner, *The Healing Process,* August 29, 1924, London.

and no longer feel the heaviness of earth. The soul feels as though united with a cosmos of music and enters into a kind of dream or "intoxication."

In the image of the stepmother who is forced to dance in red-hot shoes until she falls down dead, on the other hand, the dream of dancing has become a nightmare and the intoxication a consuming agitation that leads to death. In such a dance, the sickness of the body and the fever of the soul burn till they are burnt out. The demonic self (the stepmother) is overcome and perishes, while the newly mature soul (Snow White) can unite with her higher self (the King's son) and become a young and happy queen.

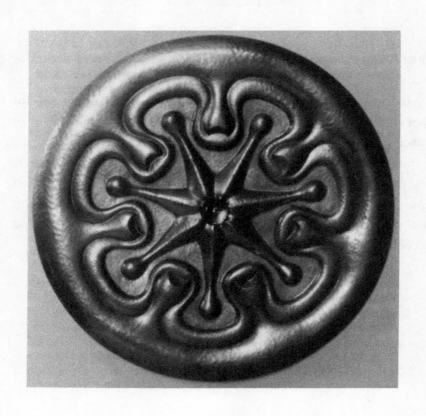

Jupiter Seal

MERCURY AS A REMEDY: "THE MASTER THIEF"

One day an old man and his wife were sitting in front of a miserable house resting a while from their work. Suddenly a splendid carriage with four black horses came driving up, and a richly dressed man descended from it. The peasant stood up, went to the great man, and asked what he wanted and in what way he could be useful to him? The stranger stretched out his hand to the old man and said, "I want nothing but to enjoy for once a country dish; cook me some potatoes, in the way you always have them, and then I will sit down at your table and eat them with pleasure."

The peasant smiled and said, "You are a count or a prince, or perhaps even a duke; noble gentlemen often have such fancies, but you shall have your wish."

The wife went into the kitchen and began to wash and rub the potatoes and to make them into balls, as they are eaten by country-folk. While she was busy with this work, the peasant said to the stranger, "Come into my garden with me for a while. I have more to do there." He had dug some holes in the garden and now wanted to plant some trees in them.

"Have you no children," asked the stranger, "who could help you with your work?"

"No," answered the peasant, "I had a son, it is true, but it is long since he went out into the world. He was a ne'er-do-well, sharp and knowing, but he would learn nothing and was full of bad tricks. Finally, he ran away from me, and since then I have heard nothing of him."

The old man took a young tree, put it in a hole, drove in a post beside it, and when he had shoveled in some earth and had trampled it firmly down, he tied the stem of the tree above, below, and in the middle, fast to the post by a rope of straw. "But tell me," said the stranger, "why you don't tie that crooked knotted tree, which is lying in the corner there, bent down almost to the ground, to a post also that it may grow straight, as well as these?"

The old man smiled and said, "Sir, you speak according to your knowledge it is easy to see that you are not familiar with gardening. That tree there is old and misshapen; no one can make it straight now. Trees must be trained while they are young."

"That is how it was with your son," said the stranger. "If you had trained him while he was still young, he would not have run away; now he, too, must have grown hard and misshapen."

"Truly it is a long time since he went away," replied the old man, "he must have changed."

"Would you know him again if he were to come to you?" asked the stranger.

"Hardly by his face," replied the peasant, "but he has a mark about him—a birthmark on his shoulder that looks like a bean." When he had said that the stranger pulled off his coat, bared his shoulder, and showed the peasant the bean.

"Good God!" cried the old man, "You are really my son!" With this, love for his child stirred in his heart. "But," he added, "how can you be my son? You have become a great lord and live in wealth and luxury. How have you contrived to do that?"

"Ah, father," answered the son, "the young tree was bound to no post and has grown crooked. Now it is too old and will never be straight again. How have I got all that? I have become a thief, but do not be alarmed, I am a Master Thief. For me there are neither locks nor bolts; whatsoever I desire is mine. Do not imagine that I steal like a common thief. I take only some of the superfluity of the rich. Poor people are safe; I would rather give to them than take anything from them. It is the same with anything that I can have without trouble, cunning, and dexterity—I never touch it."

"Alas, my son," said the father, "it still does not please me; a thief is still a thief. I tell you it will end badly."

He took him to his mother, and when she heard that was her son, she wept for joy, but when he told her that he had become a master thief, two streams flowed down over her face. At length she said, "Even if he has become a thief, he is still my son, and my eyes have beheld him once more."

They sat down to table, and once again with his parents he ate the wretched food he had not eaten for so long. The father said, "If our lord, the count up there in the castle, learns who you are and the trade you follow he will not take you in his arms and cradle you as he did when he held you at the font, but will cause you to swing from a halter."

"Be easy, father, he will do me no harm, for I understand my trade. I will go to him myself this very day."

When evening drew near, the master thief seated himself in his carriage and drove to the castle. The count received him civilly, for he took him for a distinguished man. When, however, the stranger made himself known, the count turned pale and was silent for quite some time. At length he said, "You are my godson, and on that account mercy shall take the place of justice, and I will deal leniently with you. Since you pride yourself on being a master thief, I will put your art to the proof. But if you do not stand the test, you must marry the rope maker's daughter, and the croaking of the raven must be your music on that occasion."

"Lord Count," answered the master thief, "Think of three things, as difficult as you like, and if I do not perform your tasks, do with me what you will."

The count reflected for some minutes and said, "Well, then, first you shall steal the horse I keep for my own riding out of the stable. Next you shall steal the sheet from beneath the bodies of my wife and myself while we sleep and without our observing it—and the wedding ring of my wife as well. Third and last, you shall steal the parson and clerk from the church. Mark what I am saying, for your life depends on it."

The master thief went to the nearest town, where he bought the clothes of an old peasant woman and put them on. Then he stained his face brown and painted wrinkles on it so that no one could recognize him. Then he filled a small cask with old Hungarian wine, in which was mixed a powerful sleeping potion. He put the cask into a basket, which he put on his back and walked with slow and tottering steps toward the count's castle.

It was already dark when he arrived. He sat on a stone in the courtyard and began to cough like an asthmatic old woman and rubbed his hands together as if he were cold. In front of the door of the stable some soldiers were lying round a fire; one of them observed the woman and called out to her, "Come nearer, old mother, and warm yourself beside us. After all, you have no bed for the night and must take one where you can find it."

The old woman tottered up to them, begged them to lift the basket from her back, and sat down beside them at the fire. "What have you got in your little cask, old lady?" asked one.

"A good mouthful of wine," she answered. "I live by trade, for money and fair words I am quite ready to let you have a glass."

"Let us have it here, then," said the soldier, and when he had tasted one glass he said, "When wine is good, I like another glass." He had another poured out for himself, and the rest followed his example.

"Hallo, comrades," cried one of them to those who were in the stable, "here is an old goody who has wine that is as old as herself; take a drink; it will warm your stomachs far better than our fire."

The old woman carried her cask into the stable. One of the soldiers had seated himself on the saddled riding horse, another held its bridle in his hand, and a third laid hold of its tail. She poured out as much as they wanted until the spring ran dry.

It was not long before the bridle fell from the hand of the one, and he fell and began to snore; the other left hold of the tail, lay down and snored even louder. The one who was sitting in the saddle remained sitting, but bent his head almost to the horse's neck as he slept and blew with his mouth like the bellows of a forge.

The soldiers outside had been asleep for a long time already and were lying motionless on the ground as if dead. When the master thief saw that he had succeeded, he gave the first a rope in his hand instead of the bridle and a wisp of straw to the other who had been holding the tail. But what was he to do with the one sitting on the horse's back? He did not want to throw him down, for he might have awakened and cried out.

He had a good idea. He unbuckled the girths of the saddle, tied a couple of ropes that were hanging on a ring on the wall fast to the saddle, and drew the sleeping rider up into the air on it, then he twisted the rope round the posts and tied it fast. He soon unloosed the horse from the chain, but if he had ridden over the stony pavement of the yard they would have heard the noise in the castle. So he wrapped the horse's hoofs in old rags, led him carefully out, leapt upon him, and galloped off.

When day broke, the master galloped to the castle on the stolen horse. The count had just gotten up and was looking out the window. "Good morning, Sir Count," he cried to him, "here is the horse, which I got safely out of the stable! Just look, how beautifully your soldiers are lying there asleep. And if you will only go into the stable, you will see how comfortable your watchers have made it for themselves."

The count could not help laughing and said, "For once you have succeeded, but things won't go so well the second time. I warn you that, if you come before me as a thief, I will handle you as I would any thief."

When the countess went to bed that night, she closed her hand with the wedding ring tightly together, and the count said, "All the doors are locked and bolted, I will keep awake and wait for the thief; but if he gets in by the window, I will shoot him."

The master thief, however, went in the dark to the gallows, cut down a poor sinner who was hanging there, and carried him on his back to the castle. Then he set a ladder up to the bedroom, put the dead body on his shoulders, and began to climb. When he had gotten so high that the head of the dead man showed at the window, the count, who was watching in his bed, fired a pistol at him, and immediately the master let the poor sinner fall down, and hid himself in one corner.

The night was sufficiently moonlit that the master thief could distinctly see the count climbing out the window onto to the ladder. He came down, carried the dead body into the garden, and began to dig a hole in which to lay it.

Now, thought the thief, *the favorable moment has come.* He stole nimbly out of his corner and climbed the ladder right into the countess's bedroom. "Dear wife," he began in the count's voice, "the thief is dead, but, after all, he is my godson and has been more an incorrigible rascal than a villain. I will not put him to open shame. Besides, I am sorry for the parents. I will bury him myself before daybreak in the garden so that the thing may not be known. So give me the sheet; I will wrap up the body in it and bury him like a dog." The countess gave him the sheet.

"I tell you what," continued the thief, "I have a fit of magnanimity on me; give me the ring, too; the unhappy man risked his life for it, so he may take it with him into his grave."

She would not disagree with the count, and although she did it unwillingly she drew the ring from her finger and gave it to him. The thief made off with both these things and reached home safely before the count had finished his work of burying in the garden.

What a long face the count had when the master thief came next morning and brought with him the sheet and ring. "Are you a wizard?" he asked. "Who has fetched you out of the grave in which I myself laid you and brought you to life again?"

"You did not bury me," said the thief, "but the poor sinner from the gallows." He told him exactly how everything had happened, and the count was forced to admit to him that he was a clever, crafty thief.

"But you have not yet reached the end," he added. "You still have the third task to perform, and if you do not succeed in that all is for nothing." The master smiled and returned no answer.

When night had fallen, the master thief went to the village church with a long sack on his back, a bundle under his arms, and a lantern in his hand. In the sack were some crabs and in the bundle short wax candles. He sat down in the churchyard, took out a crab, and stuck a wax candle on his back. Then he lit the small light, placed the crab on the ground, and let it creep about. He took a second out of the sack, and treated it in the same way, and so on until the last one was out of the sack.

With this, he put on a long black garment that looked like a monk's cowl and stuck a gray beard on his chin. Finally, when he was unrecognizable, he took the sack in which the crabs had been, went into the church, and ascended the pulpit. The clock in the tower was just striking twelve. When the last stroke had sounded, he cried with a loud and piercing voice, "Hearken, sinful people, the end of all things has come! The last day is at hand! Hearken! Hearken! Whosoever wishes to go to Heaven with me must creep into the sack. I am Peter, who opens and shuts the gate of Heaven. Behold how the dead outside there in the churchyard are wandering about collecting their bones. Come, come, and creep into the sack; the world is about to be destroyed!"

The cry echoed through the whole village. The parson and clerk, who lived nearest the church, heard it first, and when they saw the lights moving about the churchyard, they observed that something unusual was going on and went into the church. They listened to the sermon for a while, and then the clerk nudged the parson and said, "It would not be amiss if we were to use the opportunity together and, before the dawning of the last day, find an easy way of getting to Heaven."

"To tell the truth," answered the parson, "that is what I myself have been thinking, so if you are inclined we will set out on our way."

"Yes," answered the clerk, "but you, the pastor, have the precedence. I will follow." So the parson went first and ascended the pulpit, where the master opened his sack. The parson crept in first, and then the clerk. The master immediately tied up the sack tightly, seized it by the middle, and dragged it down the pulpit steps. Whenever the heads of the two fools bumped on the steps, he cried, "We are going over the mountains."

Then he drew them through the village in the same way, and when they were passing through puddles he cried, "Now we are going through wet clouds." And finally, when he was dragging them up the steps of the castle, he cried, "Now we are on the steps of Heaven, and will soon be in the outer court."

When he reached the top, he pushed the sack into the pigeon house, and when the pigeons fluttered about, he said, "Hark how glad the angels are, and how they are flapping their wings!" Then he bolted the door upon them and went away.

Next morning, he went to the count and told him that he had performed the third task, as well, and had carried the parson and clerk out of the church. "Where have you left them?" asked the lord.

"They are lying upstairs in a sack in the pigeon house and imagine that they are in Heaven."

The count went up and convinced himself that the master had told the truth. Once he had delivered the parson and clerk from their captivity, he said, "You are an arch thief and have won your wager. For once, you escape with a whole skin, but see that you leave my land, for if ever you set foot on it again, you may count on your elevation to the gallows."

The arch-thief took leave of his parents, once more went forth into the wide world, and no one has ever heard of him since.[1]

---

1   Source: http://ebooks.adelaide.edu.au/g/grimm/g86h/chapter193.html (revised).

Mercury, the Metal

In this chapter we take up a tale that appears to fit in poorly with
the others in our study. The initial impression is of a farce, a droll
tale. Appropriately, the metal for which this tale serves as a background is also "uncharacteristic" in its properties, presenting a clear
contrast to the other planetary metals. Taken together, the events in
"The Master Thief" and the specific qualities of the metal mercury
will help us grasp the character of the planet Mercury and the corresponding metal process.

The term *Mercury,* from Latin *Mercurius,* applies both to the
metal once known as *quicksilver* and to the associated planet. As we
penetrate into the idiosyncrasies of this metal and the farcical motifs
of the tale, we shall discover, as we did with the other fairy tales,
that a deep truth and wisdom lie hidden in them.[2] The many and
seemingly contradictory facets of the Mercury dynamic then become
understandable, and we are no longer puzzled why such divergent
groups as doctors, merchants, tradespeople... and thieves... once all
claimed Mercury as their patron deity. Moreover, we gain a new perspective on the therapeutic use of potentized mercury preparations.

First, some of the stranger properties of metallic mercury. It is the
only metal that occurs as a liquid, the state in which all metals exist
before they solidify. Because of this, it unites two opposing properties
in itself; when encountering an obstacle, mercury breaks into countless tiny droplets, but when the droplets come into even the slightest
contact they instantly reunite as a whole. Thus mercury bears forces of
both dissolution and unification. These two opposite properties might
also be called "releasing" and "binding." Hence, just as water dis-
solves salt, mercury is able to dissolve other metals in itself, yet it is

---

2   Paul Paede has connected mercury with the Grimms' tale "The Spirit in
     the Bottle." The study was published in the *Beiträge zu einer Erweiterung
     der Heilkunst,* no. 4, 1970, Stuttgart. In her book *Metallfunktionstypen
     in Psychologie und Medizin* (Types of Metal Function in Psychology and
     Medicine), Alla Selawry cites the Master Thief as an embodiment of the
     Mercury type.

also able to unite with most other metals in solid amalgams. Metals that neither dissolve in mercury nor combine with it are few—chiefly earthy metals like iron. In this sense Mercury leads a genuine "double life"; it is able to enter into affinity relationships with opposites, but also to release them. Hence the term *mercurial* applies to a process that stands between two poles while maintaining a relationship to both.

The Motifs and Mood of the Tale; the Mercury Process

No one who reads "The Master Thief" can help smiling, perhaps even laughing at moments. The tale creates a genuinely humorous mood, and humor is liberating. This, in fact, is a specific Mercury characteristic. One way that Mercury expresses its liberating quality is by exposing the transitory nature of things—how quickly they pass, how easily they change. With humor, things that want to take up permanent residence in the soul are recognized for what they are—transient and trivial. Mercury helps us realize that, in the end, even the most sublime experience is only a stage in an unending development. The Mercurial is the fluid, mobile, changeable element in the great life of the cosmos, and the mood of our story matches it well; it is the light-hearted tale of a master in the art of thievery.

The plot of the story is extraordinarily fluid, full of changes and surprises, constantly introducing unexpected and implausible turns. But the Master Thief proves more than a match for the most outlandish predicaments. Like the Mercury process that unites the two forces of binding and releasing, the Master Thief continually manages to slip into new and often diametrically opposed roles. His double life is based on the gift of transformation, which he puts to use at critical moments and so remains uncatchable. With sovereign ease he passes all the tests that the count sets him. On the other hand, the subtler lessons that he himself offers are not understood by the count, who wishes to persist in his accustomed world, where things remain graspable and simple. Because the Master Thief poses a threat to this condition, he is expelled from the land.

With these introductory thoughts we have merely sketched out the correspondences between the tale and the metal process. Now we can proceed to a more detailed study that will reveal the full depth—and also the ambiguity—of this tale.

The Mercury Character

First let us take a closer look at the general connection between Mercury and "The Master Thief." In the soul realm the Mercury process is the agent of humor, liberating us with the recognition that nothing is immutable in this transitory world. By keeping everything in flux, it banishes heaviness, hardness, and fear. The true Mercury type has a light, perhaps even happy-go-lucky manner, and a buoyant, sanguine temperament. Such is the Master Thief himself, who is mercurial in every facet of his character. A master in the art of disguise and transformation, there is no role he cannot slip into. He is effervescent life and exuberant motion; his whole being radiates wit and humor. In describing him we describe the character of Mercury, and vice versa.

The Mercury Process and Transformation

Turning now to the three tests that the count poses the Master Thief, we come to a natural question: What is the significance of this quality of three? Let us attempt an interpretation. As his first test, the Master Thief must steal the count's personal steed—a horse so well guarded that stealing it seems an impossibility. This creature is his absolute property, and under no circumstances may it be taken from him! In this tale the horse can be recognized as a symbol of reason and independent thinking;[3] so to restate this image, the count regards his reason, his power of thought, as his inalienable property. He considers himself the master of his mental faculties, but he is wrong; the Master Thief has no difficulty putting the entire horse

---

3   Steiner, "Über das zehnblättrige Buch; fragmentarische Notizen nach einem Vortrag gehalten am 3.4.1905 in Berlin," *Beiträge zur Rudolf Steiner Gesamtausgabe*, no. 32, Christmas 1970.

guard to sleep. In spite of all the count's precautions, his horse is stolen and led away; reason and independent thinking can be distracted onto other paths; they can "escape" their owner. In this way the Master Thief demonstrates to the count that he cannot be considered the master—let alone the owner—of his mental powers if he is so easily deprived of them. In fact it is the Master Thief who is the true master of the powers of reason and thinking. And he is master not only in this realm—the nerve-sense system—but also in the rhythmic and metabolic systems, as the two following tests show.

The Mercury Process and the Capacity for Meeting

The second test that the Master Thief must pass relates to the rhythmic system, which connects the nerve-sense system and metabolic-limb system. By allowing these two poles to interweave, it is able to join together and harmoniously unify their opposite natures. Joining and union are indicated in the tale by the ring and the bed sheet. The wedding ring symbolizes the conjoining of two human beings, while the sheet of the marriage bed points to their state of union. Yet as the second test shows, these seemingly so fixed and permanent things can be undone with playful ease by the Master Thief. And if the count was still able to laugh after his first defeat, now he is perplexed and begins to wonder if the Master Thief is a wizard.

Things get dramatic in this second test. The count takes out his pistol and shoots the supposed thief, protecting his wedding ring and bed sheet as if his own life were at stake. The count was willing to let others guard his horse, but now he lies in wait himself. In this behavior we recognize a personification of the ordinary, everyday self when it feels directly threatened. An attack on the center, the rhythmic system, represents a mortal threat to the self, and so it is not surprising that this test becomes a matter of life and death. We are no longer dealing with a prank; there is nothing farcical in the dramatic action here; it could very quickly turn to tragedy.

The ring is also an image of the self-enclosed soul.[4] It may be that this ring is made of gold, and gold in itself represents wisdom; yet when gold is made into a ring, this can be taken as an indication that the wisdom aspect is shut out and has turned into self-seeking. Wisdom was once united with the world and served the whole. As the human being awakens to personhood, our striving begins to center on ourselves and enters the realm of self-seeking. Thus the wedding ring can be regarded not only as a symbol of the wholeness of two united souls, but also as an image for the tendency of every soul to close itself off, to create boundaries and lose the capacity for real meeting. The coming together of two people in marriage can mean that one seeks in the other what he or she is missing and wishes complemented by the other. From this perspective, marriage may ultimately be based on the longing to find in the other a mirror of one's own complete self. In such a case no true meeting with one's partner is possible. When we need the other for self-affirmation and use that person as a mirror of our own perfection, we are unable to recognize the individual. We are deceiving ourselves and will be disappointed.

This deception is the central motif of the second test. The count is deceived when he takes the corpse for the Master Thief and shoots at it. His wife too is deceived, when she takes the Master Thief for her husband and unthinkingly hands over the bed sheet and the ring to him. So it is that the Master Thief passes this test as well with ease, and this cannot help but be disturbing to the count.

The Mercury Process and Release

Now what about the third test? As in the two preceding tests, the Mercury process manifests itself here as a process of dissolution. This time, however, the dissolution applies to the metabolic-limb system. The cosmic-spiritual is acting here on the level of substance, not of process. The metabolism harbors the forces that strive toward

---

4   Steiner, "Notizen zum öffentlichen Vortrag vom 1. April 1908 in Stockholm," *Nachrichten der Rudolf Steiner Nachlaßverwaltung*, no. 22, Michaelmas 1968, Dornach.

release, as opposed to the forces of "fixation" found in the nerve-sense system. Let us explore this opposition. Through our senses we perceive the world around us, but primarily its forms and structures, not its substances; these are rejected. With the sensory forces, the forces of thought above all, we strive to take hold of the spiritual content of the world. Through them comes the "in-formation" that we eagerly take in—according to our interests and disposition—to come to an understanding of the world and its phenomena. The metabolism works in a completely different way. Here substances are taken in, while their forms and structures are rejected. The substances are completely broken down and drawn into a new connection with the organism. So here, the organism unites with the spirituality of the world not through form but through substance, or rather through its breaking-down. And the forces that bring about this dissolution are inflammatory forces, sulfuric forces. They are forces that cannot wait, that hunger to take in this spirituality. At all costs they will unite with the spirituality of the substances. All the metabolic processes are based on this powerful hunger to unite, to merge completely our own spirituality with the spirituality of the substances.

Thus the contrast; the upper pole of the human being is disposed to receive passively. The spiritual content of the world "in-forms" us and we preserve it, fixing it in our minds. But in the metabolism the organism unites actively with the spiritual forces of the world around it by decomposing its substances, transforming and assimilating them in a continual process of de- and re-construction that releases them from their previous material form. It is from this particular aspect of the metabolism that we can look at the third test. The hunger, indeed the greed, of the parson and the clerk—those two immature "servants of God"—for effortless and immediate redemption can be understood as an imaginative expression of the hunger of the metabolic-limb system for the cosmic-spiritual. Their desire blinds them to reality, and the Master Thief is able to put this blindness to good use. We are presented with a parody of redemption.

The Master Thief's Lessons and the Mercury Process

To review, in the first test the Master Thief befuddles the heads of the guards and puts them to sleep; in the second he poses as the count to the latter's wife; and in the third he plays with the desire for redemption. In all three tests the Master Thief casts seemingly well-established forms into disorder, and all for the sake of showing that nothing is certain and indissoluble. This "Master" takes nothing for his own benefit; his masterpieces of thievery are each intended as warnings and lessons. His demonstrations are intended to teach the count—and all of us with him—that as human beings we can never be wakeful enough in regard to our rational mind and sense impressions, that we should not rely on sensations and feelings, and that our yearning for redemption must be tempered by patient waiting. Thus the tests are lessons on the spiritual path and point to the dangers that meet us on it. On such a path it easily happens that all certainty disappears and every order seems threatened. Yet the confusion and disorder caused by the Master make it possible for something new to arise.

The Mercury process—the Master—is the mediator, the one who loosens old ties, preparing us to find our higher Selves. The activity of the Master, who casts doubt on the old external order and exposes it to ridicule, makes room for inner change and growth so that the new can take form. Not even the resurrection of the dead is spared from the Master's devices when it is useful to his purposes. He parodies what is held sacred, touching on an area that belongs to the most intimate layers of the human soul, the longing to participate in the eternal sphere. Yet in the third test the Master shows just how quickly this longing leads to self-deception. In this way he leads us to ponder: What exactly is the eternal "I," the sacred, divine spark in the human being?

Mercury is the one whom the Greeks called "thrice-great," Hermes Trismegistos, ruler over the three soul realms of thinking, feeling, and willing. In these three realms it is not the personal self that exercises power, as might be assumed. No, the Mercury process points clearly to a different truth, one that can initially cause great insecurity and loss of self-confidence. Yet out of this instability a power can develop that leads toward finding the true self and true self-confidence. These lie on another level, on the level where we seek the eternal spiritual nature of our own individuality behind the transitory. It is here that the real human "I" is at work.

In the tale, this level is not reached. The count—the everyday self—cannot tolerate the lack of security; he clings to the old order. Therefore he banishes the Master from the land without delay, never to return again. The self is still too attached to the transitory, and the higher "I" is still too weak and immature to recognize the lessons.

Mercurius *as a Remedy*

Mercury in its various compounds is an important remedy both in homeopathy and in anthroposophic medicine. The disease pictures for which *Mercurius* preparations are therapeutically effective can be recognized as Imaginations in the tale chosen here. Each of these disease pictures reflects either an excessive or a deficient Mercury process. Now we shall describe the disease pictures and then show their connections to the tale. First let us look at the manifestations of these deviations on the soul plane.

The Disease Picture on the Soul Plane

The healthy Mercury type is a slim and agile limbed person with a sanguine temperament. When the Mercury process is out of balance, one of two different extremes results; on the one hand the type who seems "possessed" by Mercury—the fidgety smart aleck in need of constant change; on the other hand the type who seems to have been abandoned by Mercury—the unintelligent, awkward, and isolated individual. With an excessive Mercury process, the patient's soul life becomes unbalanced and displays exaggerated, uncontrolled reactions. He is rushed, restless, and irritable. When this picture reaches a pathological stage, it bears the name of *Erethism mercurialis*. Here the agility, speed and quick-wittedness characteristic of the Master Thief have taken on an exaggerated life of their own. The agility has turned into fidgetiness, the speed to haste, and the quick-wittedness to distraction.

For the excessive Mercury process that leads to pathologies such as *Erethism mercurialis,* effective remedies include *Mercurius vivus naturalis* in mid-potencies, D 10 to D 15, or *Mercurius* as a vegetized metal—potentized by the plant, to so speak—in the form of *Bryophyllum mercurio cultum* D2 or D3. For the opposite picture— the too weak Mercury process—we need only reverse the condition described above and the symptoms will stand before us in complete clarity. Instead of agitation we find an empty-headed nature. The Mercury-abandoned individual is dull, clumsy, and highly averse to leaving his habitual sphere. This patient characteristically exhibits sluggishness on all levels. Constitutionally he is prone to lymphatic abnormalities, which can be effectively treated with *Mercurius vivus naturalis* in low potencies (e.g., D3 to D6).

Mercurius *Preparations and their Organ Associations*

The primary physical pathologies for which *Mercurius* is used therapeutically are mucosal affections and diseases of the lymphatic and glandular system.[5] In regard to the mucosae, mercury has a special connection to those of the digestive tract, particularly the oral region and the large intestine—that is, the beginning and end of the digestive tract. Mercury preparations have little connection to the central portion, stomach, and small intestine. They act on the portions of the digestive apparatus that have to do with the preparatory breakdown and the conclusion of digestion—the thickening and solidification. These two areas stand at opposite poles, but in both the mouth and in the large intestine the liquid is present alongside the

---

5   Manfred Weckenmann, "Die Beziehung zwischen empirisch und
     geisteswissenschaftlich gewonnenen Arzneimittelbildern von Quecksilber,"
     Der Merkurstab 1, Stuttgart, 1988.

solid. The area to which *Mercurius* has no clear relation is the purely liquid phase, where the actual absorption of nutrients takes place. In the large intestine we also see a type of peristalsis that does not occur in its preceding sections—*antiperstalsis,* by which the intestinal content is pushed back toward the appendix, thus reversing the previous order of the digestive realm. The function of reverse peristalsis is to enable thorough thickening.

Intestinal Peristalsis and Thinking

It is important and instructive to note the close relationship between the large intestine and mobility of thought.[6] Whatever happens in the lower pole of the human organism—the metabolic-limb system—always has a correspondence in the upper pole, the nerve-sense system. The ancient esoteric law, "as above, so below," applies not only to the macrocosm (the world), but also to the microcosm (the human being). The fact that intestinal digestive processes correlate with certain thought patterns can be empirically observed in patients who take psychopharmaceutical drugs such as antidepressants. Not only is their thinking retarded and less flexible than normal, but they also suffer frequently from constipation.[7] It is evident that there is a connection between mental agility and the digestive process in the large intestine.

When the opposite occurs, when mental life becomes inconstant, rushed, and "greedy," then the lower pole exhibits a tendency to diarrhea. The large intestine is irritated and cannot thicken the stool. What is missing is the ability to wait and take back. The parallel to this in our tale is seen in the third test, when the parson and the clerk fall into the Master Thief's trap, caught by their greed for redemption. They seem to experience earthly existence as a burden that they

---

6   Steiner, *Harmony of the Creative Word,* Nov. 2, 1923; Steiner, "Aufzeichnungen zur Medizin," from Steiner's notebooks and loose notes, "Nachrichten der Rudolf Steiner Nachlaßverwaltung," Dornach, no. 20, Christmas 1967.

7   R. Wagner, "Stuhlunregeläßigkeiten," *Therapiewoche* 36, p. 498, 1986.

would be glad to be released from, the sooner the better. To translate this medically, the organism experiences the unusable content of the intestine as a burden of which it wishes to be speedily relieved. It cannot wait for this to happen in its own good time.

Mercurius *and Sore Throat*

Now we turn to the region of the organism where the process of digestion begins: the mouth and pharynx. *Mercurius* preparations are in fact the most important remedies for the treatment of pharyngitis, so we must look closely at this ailment from the perspective of mercury. In pharyngitis the cervical lymph nodes are swollen and inflamed. The patient can swallow only with pain. This is not just a symptom of the ailment; it is its signature. "I can't swallow" as a physical symptom is frequently connected with "I won't swallow" as a soul attitude. The patient resists experiences that affect him too strongly or threaten his worldview. The latter has taken form out of his experiences and memories and has become firmly entrenched in his consciousness. He is so comfortable with it that he cannot face new steps in inner development or urgent external changes. He wants to hold on to the familiar and refuses to "swallow" the new. For fear of losing what is known and comforting, his consciousness resists the inner maturation process. Amid these conflicting forces a state of tension develops, causing congestion in the etheric body. At this point it takes only one additional stressor, such as an elevated risk of infection or a chill, to transform the blockage into manifest illness. The patient develops an inflammation of the throat—pharyngitis or tonsillitis.

Polarity and Correspondence of Colitis and Pharyngitis

As we contrast the two diseases—inflammation of the large intestine and that of the tonsillar ring—their polarities and commonalities emerge with clarity. In the case of colitis, the patient's soul holds an overly powerful (though generally unconscious) desire for spiritualization, for release. His thinking tends to move in a wish-ful, metaphysical direction and would gladly shut out the realities and troubles of everyday existence. This is a kind of escapism. Such a person is unable to wait calmly and let things develop at their own pace—including his own development and maturation.[8]

The pharyngitis patient has exactly the opposite inner disposition. He is dominated by fear of change, fear of losing what is familiar and known. All feelings that rise too close to his conscious awareness meet with resistance in him—in particular when they would require any deep transformation in his own soul. What these two disease ten-dencies have in common is how difficult it is for the patients to come to terms with real life; at bottom, they lack a healthy self-confidence. They are afraid they are no match for the obstacles and tend either toward inner resistance and denial or toward escapism and hopeless-ness. Therefore they lack the power to grow and mature through fac-ing their subjective, inner deficiencies or the objective, external ones. Life-mastery requires accepting what cannot be changed as well as dealing effectively with what is unacceptable. In these patients, how-ever, wishful thinking and fear of confronting their inner world gen-erally get in the way.

Fairy-Tale Imaginations as Disease Pictures

Let us now briefly revisit the tale and attempt to relate it to the under-standing we have developed of these pathologies. The Master Thief's third test offers an illustration of blind desire—the desire to escape as easily and quickly as possible from the painstaking work and mundane duties of everyday existence. This desire makes a person blind even to his own reason. In light of such an interpretation, the third test can be connected imaginatively to the pathology that manifests as colitis.

---

8   Rainer Sandweg, "Zur Psychodynamik und Therapie chronisch-entzündli-cher Darmerkrankungen," *Praxis der Psychotherapie und Psychosomatik* 34, 1989, pp. 73–81; Klaus Fischer und Sybille Großhans, "Colitis ulcerosa- und Morbus Crohn-Patienten in psychischer und biographischer Hinsicht–Eine Studie," *Merkurstab*, Stuttgart, 4–5, 1989.

The first test, in contrast, portrays a soul disposition that clings to the mindset and the worldview it feels at home with. The horse (the patient's thinking) is tied up tight—as in a spasm—by the tail and bridle; moreover, one guard sits astride it to avoid the slightest chance of its being lost. Here we discern the soul attitude of the pharyngitis patient, who cannot or will not give up ideas he has grown attached to and rejects everything new. Such a patient must be "anaesthetized" before he can let go of his accustomed thought patterns. This is in fact what happens in pharyngitis, when (as so often) it is associated with flu; the patient experiences a dimming of consciousness.

Opening the Center, Perceiving the Other, and Self-Knowledge

We have explored the upper and lower Mercury process by relating the first and third tests to corresponding disease pictures. Now let us turn to the middle Mercury process. The tale depicts this process in the tricks by which the Master Thief steals the wedding ring and the bed sheet. From the Mercury perspective, the middle realm is always an area of encounter and exchange. This is where we recognize the true spiritual being of another person, and where we can experience our own identity. This balancing center, with its warmth of heart, enables us to perceive and recognize the Other as an independent spiritual individuality, and at the same time to experience fully our own Self. It is an apparent paradox, but perception of the other, the experience of "you," is always connected with genuine self-recognition. The two forms of knowledge are mutually conditioned.

This phenomenon is not limited to the soul plane; in fact, corresponding processes take place on the biological plane as well. The most relevant example for us is the lymphatic system, which (as we have seen) has a special connection to the Mercury process. Countless new insights in the area of immunology—especially regarding the function of the lymphocytes—reveal just how complex, how many-layered, are the processes involved in the recognition of self and non-self. The lymphocytes must first "surrender" to foreign influences and unite with them before they are able to perceive them as incompatible with the life of the organism. We will explore this aspect in greater detail when we consider Hodgkin's disease.

Our sense of self initially requires reinforcement—this lies in the nature of self-awareness. The reactions of the other person are experienced as a mirror for our sense of self. In self-infatuation we believe we recognize the other, but we only perceive the unconscious projection of our own self. In other words, we experience the other as a complement, a "completion" of our self. Falling passionately in love, for example, can mean becoming blind with love. What is it that one falls in love with in such cases? It is really that part of the other that affirms our own sense of self. Great disappointments are inevitable when the whole enterprise began with such a fundamental error.

Appropriately, the second test in the tale deals with the obstacles to knowing oneself and recognizing the other. The count and his wife both fail to recognize whom they are dealing with. The count takes a corpse for the Master Thief and shoots it; the countess takes the Master Thief for her husband and hands over the ring and bed sheet to him. As we discovered, the ring and the bed sheet represent an egocentric condition of self-satisfaction, so they must be lost by falling into the hands of the Master Thief. Thus, all the encounters in this test are based on illusion and error. No opening of the self and no real perception of the other have taken place. By falling prey to such delusions, the count and the countess show that they do not really know themselves; as we have discussed, recognition of the other is always contingent on self-recognition.

As with all the fairy tales chosen in our study to illuminate hidden connections, the images relate not only to the psychological but equally to the biological plane; the physiological, pathological, and in this case especially the immunological. Let us examine the second test from this point of view.

The Hodgkin's Patient and Mercurius

When we consider Hodgkin's disease (Hodgkin's lymphoma) on the background of the preceding discussion, we discover correspondences with the second test. Hodgkin's patients can be described as follows; they are generally harmoniously built, often blond with delicate skin and rosy complexion. They combine an alert interest for the world around them with unusually high sensitivity to outer and inner experiences. Middle-aged men are more frequently affected than women and also have a poorer prognosis. Patients are notable for disturbances in the immune system with abnormalities of the globulins, manifested in non-rejection of foreign skin transplants, for example; the immune system allows itself to be tricked. In contrast to the clean medical history of many cancer patients, among Hodgkin's patients one often notes a tendency to repeated inflammations, particularly of the upper respiratory passages and the tonsils.

In the soul realm, Hodgkin's patients display a striking sensitivity and vulnerability along with pronounced extraversion. Patients are highly impressionable but lack sufficient inner stability. They enter without difficulty into the life around them but do not really meet it.[9] Rather, it seems they need it only for self-confirmation, and if they do not receive this—if they encounter criticism, for example—they feel deeply hurt. Essentially, they need the other only as a mirror to reflect themselves. Hence, the paradox—that in spite of their sensitivity, despite their interest in the other, Hodgkin's patients remain without an inner connection to the other. Therefore, at the age when others enter deeper relationships—when they seek to discover which man or which woman might be the right partner, when they consider how to form this relationship so as to grow and mature in it—these vulnerable patients encounter serious problems and crises. And these often bring the illness to manifestation.

---

9   Rita Leroi, "Wesen der Hodgin-Erkrankung," *Mitteilungen aus der Behandlung maligner Tumoren mit Viscum album,* 2/1970 and 2/1980, Verein für Krebsforschung, Arlesheim.

Mercurius preparations are useful in treating this serious illness. Although they cannot cure it, they can mitigate its course and thus be of great help to the patient.

Lymph: Place of Encounter and Defense Post

The various functions of the lymphatic system take place in the unconscious depths of the organic process and are highly complex, as research in immunology continues to demonstrate. Here we can merely point to several fundamental aspects of this system. One of the essential functions of the lymph is to act as an organ of perception in the metabolic area. Yet this is an inward-directed perception; its ultimate function is doubtless for self-perception in the heart, where all lymph vessels lead. Unlike the blood, the lymphatic system possesses no vessels leading from the heart to the periphery, only those leading inward. And even coming from the periphery, the lymph does not initially pass through vessels; only later, after passing through the lymph glands, does it flow in definite lymphatic pathways toward the heart.

Various kinds of lymphocytes circulate in the lymph, carriers of "specific" immunity—that is, they have the capacity to recognize as foreign any substance that enters the organism by bypassing its regular functions, such as normal digestive processes, and to mount a defense against them. Such foreign substances can also be pathologically altered cells of the patients' own body (cancer cells). Significantly, this perceptual activity of the lymphocytes depends on their coming into close contact with the foreign substance. A real encounter must take place before the suspect substance can be recognized as hostile. At the same time, it is indispensable that a close connection be maintained with the body's own healthy cells, and for this too certain cells of the immune system are instrumental. It is while they are united with the foreign substances and still in connection with the cells of their own organism that lymphocytes mature. Only now are they in a position to initiate appropriate defense functions.

A predominance of the lymph over the blood is characteristic in the organism of the type that may be termed "cold-blooded." When the lymph process becomes too pronounced, it cannot sufficiently unite with the blood—"Mercury" and "Mars" cannot be reconciled—and we have the "lymphatic type": always shivering, needing warmth, as if one's blood temperature were too low. Characteristic of the lymphatic type is that one begins by letting the "non-self" in and experiencing it close up, as it were. Then lymphatic type responds with an over-reaction, an allergy. For example, in the case of a bee sting, the venom is not neutralized locally with a normal inflammatory process at the site of the sting, but is allowed to affect the whole organism, leading to a blind defense reaction, a kind of "general mobilization," or shock. The organism of the lymphatic shows a similar attitude toward nutrients; it does not break them down completely, but allows their foreign nature to enter. Then, to overcome the foreign element after all, it resorts to unusual means—excretion through the skin. The result is skin rash, eczema.

We have described several of the chief illnesses of the lymphatic type, all of them based on the same essential dynamic; what is foreign is not perceived as such and is therefore taken too deeply into the organism and must be overcome and eliminated by extraordinary means. Therefore a thorough encounter with the foreign substance, integrating what is usable and eliminating what is not, fails to take place. It is either wholly tolerated or resisted in aggressive fury.

The Encounter and Non-Self in the Hodgkin's Patient

In this patient we recognize a comparable dynamic, but transposed now to the soul plane. Here we have not a lymphatic constitution, but a "lymphatic" soul configuration; what takes place on the physiological plane in the lymphatic patient, manifesting in the swollen constitution and the scrofulous pathological symptoms, we find in the soul realm of the Hodgkin's patient. Here it is the soul that is "swollen," while the body may remain well formed. As we have shown, the Hodgkin's patient takes in external impressions deeply, just as the lymphatic organism allows foreign substances to penetrate it deeply. In both cases, the "intruders" are taken as mirrors of the self, as self-affirmation, and not recognized as foreign until they threaten to overwhelm the patient. To this, the lymphatic type responds with potentially massive allergic reactions, the Hodgkin's patient with deep vulnerability and total inner "encapsulation." In either case there is no proper encounter, no struggle, and no coming-to-terms with the foreign element.

Here again, the unmistakable parallels between the illnesses we are describing and the fairy tale can contribute significantly to our understanding of these disease pictures. Like the count who fires in blind rage at a dead man, the lymphatic patient wildly attacks foreign substances, because he lacks the necessary sureness of self-perception, the transformative warmth, and thus the ability to guide the physiological defense processes properly. And like the countess who mistakes the Master Thief for her husband, the Hodgkin's patient lacks the inner composure to recognize and process foreign impressions appropriately.

These complex relationships require closer scrutiny. The crucial element is the power by which the human "I" forms the soul sphere. When the inwardly dichotomous soul nature is permeated with "I"-power, it is possible for a true encounter with the outer world to occur. When this power is missing, the patient tends to close himself off to avoid being drawn into the inner conflict of the soul. To put it into an image, when the "I"-being—our individualized spiritual nature—closes itself off in a ring, the soul is completely permeated with selfhood; hence it remains self-centered and in everything around it seeks only reflection and affirmation of itself. But the corresponding physiological level is left to its own resources; that is, the lymphatic system receives no proper permeation and guidance from the higher members. Lacking these, it falls into chaos. From this perspective it is interesting that Hodgkin's patients do not reject foreign skin transplants while they react to normal body substances with aggressive defenses.

Thus an opening in the human middle realm, the realm of encounter, does not take place. This can occur only when the "I"-being is able to permeate the soul realm with its warmth. Then self-surrender and self-assertion hold the balance with each other; through the uniting power of the "I" they become two sides of the same activity.

The Master Thief as Master and Teacher

In the three "master strokes" we have been able to recognize the extraordinary character of this fairy tale. Through its images we were also able to reveal the specific nature of the Mercury process as it acts in the upper, middle and lower poles of the human being. By describing specific disease pictures and putting them into relationship with the corresponding fairy-tale images, we could grasp something of the mysteries of the Mercury process as it acts in the human organism.

Steiner speaks of the Mercury process as preparing for the Christ impulse.[10] Bearing this in mind, we are no longer surprised that the Master Thief in this tale is nine times referred to simply as "Master." The depth and uniqueness of this tale, and also the significance of the three "master strokes," begin to dawn on us and perhaps become understandable to a degree. We begin to recognize the fairy tale as a teaching story. Yet the attitude of the count in the tale also shows how difficult it is to accept such lessons and really learn from them. If we see the Master only as a troublemaker who turns the accepted order upside down, then we miss the point that he creates the conditions for a new and higher order that is to be won through spiritual strength. Then we are left with the ordinary self, the ordinary "I" that is not prepared to reflect on its indwelling spiritual nature, the Christ impulse, and develop this within.

---

10   Steiner, *Spiritual Beings in the Heavenly Bodies and in the Kingdoms of Nature,* Helsinki, April 13, 1912; Steiner, *Foundations of Esotericism,* Berlin, Oct. 28, 1905.

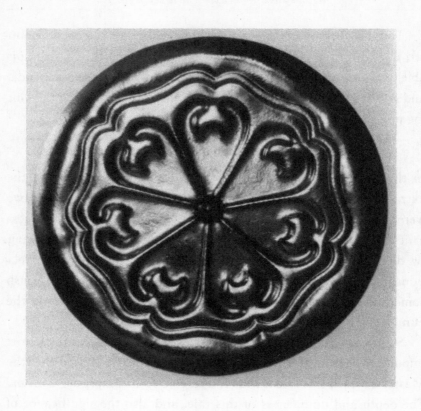

Venus Seal

SILVER AS A REMEDY: "THE SIX SWANS"

A king was once hunting in a great forest, and he chased his prey so eagerly that none of his men could follow him. As evening approached, he stopped, looked around, and saw that he was lost. He looked for a way out of the woods but could not find one. Then he saw an old woman with a bobbing head approaching him. She was a witch.

"My dear woman," he said to her, "can you show me the way through the woods?"

"Oh, yes, your majesty," she answered, "I can indeed. However, there is one condition, and if you do not fulfill it, you will never get out of these woods and will die here of hunger."

"What sort of condition is it?" asked the king.

"I have a daughter," said the old woman, "who is as beautiful as anyone you could find in all the world, and who well deserves to become your wife. If you will make her your queen, I will show you the way out of the woods."

The king was so frightened that he consented, and the old woman led him to her cottage, where her daughter was sitting by the fire. She received the king as if she had been expecting him. He saw that she was very beautiful, but in spite of this he did not like her and could not look at her without secretly shuddering.

After he had lifted the girl onto his horse, the old woman showed him the way. The king arrived again at his royal castle, where the wedding was celebrated.

The king had been married before, and he had seven children by his first wife—six boys and one girl. He loved them more than anything else in the world.

Fearing that the stepmother might not treat them well and even do them harm, he took them to a secluded castle in the middle of a forest. It was so well hidden and the way was so difficult to find that he himself would not have found it if a wise woman had not given him a ball of magic yarn. Whenever he threw it down in front of him, it would unwind itself and show him the way.

However, the king went out to his dear children so often that the queen took notice of his absence. She was curious and wanted to know what he was doing out there all alone in the woods. She gave a large sum of money to his servants, and they revealed the secret to her. They also told her about the ball of yarn that could point out the way all by itself.

She did not rest until she discovered where the king kept the ball of yarn. Then she made some little shirts of white silk. Having learned the art of witchcraft from her mother, she sewed a magic charm into each of them. Then, one day when the king had ridden out hunting, she took the little shirts and went into the woods. The ball of yarn showed her the way.

The children, seeing that someone was approaching from afar, thought that their dear father was coming to them. Full of joy, they ran to meet him. Then she threw one of the shirts over each of them, and when the shirts touched their bodies they were transformed into swans, and they flew away over the woods. The queen went home very pleased, believing that she had gotten rid of her stepchildren. However, the girl had not run out with her brothers, and the queen knew nothing about her.

The next day the king went to visit his children, but he found no one there but the girl. "Where are your brothers?" asked the king.

"Oh, dear father," she answered, "they have gone away and left me alone." Then she told him that from her window she had seen how her brothers had flown away over the woods as swans. She showed him the feathers they had dropped into the courtyard, which she had gathered up.

The king mourned, but he did not think that the queen had done this wicked deed. Fearing that the girl would be stolen away from him as well, he wanted to take her away with him, but she was afraid of her stepmother and begged the king to let her stay just this one more night in the castle in the woods. The poor girl thought, "I can no longer stay here. I will go and look for my brothers." And when night came she ran away and went straight into the woods. She walked the whole night long without stopping and the next day, as well, until she was too tired to walk any further. Then she saw a hunter's hut and went inside. She found a room with six little beds, but she did not dare to get into one of them. Instead she crawled under one of them and lay down on the hard ground where she intended to spend the night.

The Sun was about to set when she heard a rushing sound and saw six swans fly in through the window. Landing on the floor, they blew on one another and blew all their feathers off. Then their swan-skins came off just like shirts. The girl looked at them and recognized her brothers. She was happy and crawled out from beneath the bed. The brothers were no less happy to see their little sister, but their happiness did not last long. "You cannot stay here," they said to her. "This is a robbers' den. If they come home and find you, they will murder you."

"Can't you protect me?" asked the little sister.

"No," they answered. "We can take off our swan-skins for only a quarter hour each evening. We have our human forms only during that time. After that we are transformed again into swans."

Crying, the little sister said, "Can you not be redeemed?"

"Alas, no," they answered. "The conditions are too difficult. You would not be allowed to speak or to laugh for six years, and in that time you would have to sew together six little shirts from asters for us. And if a single word were to come from your mouth, all your work would be lost."

After the brothers had said this, the quarter hour was over, and they flew out the window again as swans. Nevertheless, the girl firmly resolved to redeem her brothers, even at the cost of her life.

She left the hunter's hut, went to the middle of the woods, seated herself in a tree, and there she spent the night. The next morning she went out and gathered asters and began to sew. She could not speak with anyone, and she had no desire to laugh. She sat there, looking only at her work.

After she had already spent a long time there it happened that the king of that land was hunting in those woods. His hunters came to the tree where the girl was sitting. They called to her, saying, "Who are you?" But she did not answer.

"Come down to us," they said. "We will not harm you."

She only shook her head. When they pressed her further with questions, she threw her golden necklace down to them, thinking that this would satisfy them. But they did not stop, so she then threw her belt down to them, and when this did not help, her garters, and then, one by one, everything she had on and could do without, until finally she had nothing left but her shift. The hunters, however, not letting themselves be dissuaded, climbed the tree, lifted the girl down, and took her to the king.

The king asked, "Who are you? What are you doing in that tree?" But she did not answer. He asked her in every language he knew, but she remained as speechless as a fish. Because she was so beautiful the king's heart was touched, and he fell deeply in love with her. He put his cloak around her, placed her on his horse in front of him, and took her to his castle. There he had her dressed in rich garments, and she glistened in her beauty like bright daylight, but no one could get a word from her.

At the table, he seated her by his side, and her modest manners and courtesy pleased him so much that he said, "My desire is to marry her, and no one else in the world."

A few days later they were married.

Now this king had a wicked mother who was dissatisfied with the marriage and spoke ill of the young queen. "Who knows," she said, "where the girl who cannot speak comes from? She is not worthy of a king."

A year later, after the queen had brought her first child into the world, the old woman took it away from her while she was asleep and smeared her mouth with blood. Then she went to the king and accused her of being a cannibal. The king could not believe this and would not allow anyone to harm her. She, however, sat the whole time sewing on the shirts and caring for nothing else.

The next time, she again gave birth to a beautiful boy, and her deceitful mother-in-law did the same thing again, but the king could not bring himself to believe her accusations.

He said, "She is too pious and too good to do anything like that. If she were not speechless and if she could defend herself, her innocence would come to light."

But when the old woman stole a newborn child for the third time and accused the queen, who did not defend herself with a single word, the king had no choice but to bring her to justice, and she was sentenced to die by fire.

When the day came for the sentence to be carried out, it was also the last day of the six years during which she had not been permitted to speak or to laugh, and she had thus delivered her dear brothers from the magic curse. The six shirts were finished. Only the left sleeve of the last one was missing. When she was led to the stake, she laid the shirts on her arm. Standing there, as the fire was about to be lighted, she looked around, and six swans came flying through the air. Seeing that their redemption was near, her heart leapt with joy.

The swans rushed toward her, swooping down so that she could throw the shirts over them. As soon as the shirts touched them their swan skins fell off, and her brothers stood before her in their own bodies, vigorous and handsome. However, the youngest was missing his left arm. In its place he had a swan's wing.

They embraced and kissed one another. Then the queen went to the king, who was greatly moved, and she began to speak, saying, "Dearest husband, now I may speak and reveal to you that I am innocent and falsely accused." She told him of the treacherous old woman who had taken away their three children and hidden them. Then to the king's great joy they were brought forth. As a punishment, the wicked mother-in-law was tied to the stake and burned to ashes. But the king and the queen, along with her six brothers, lived many long years in happiness and peace.[1]

~

The final tale in our study, "The Six Swans," allows us to explore the Silver process from an imaginative perspective. Since this process is connected with the last planetary realm that the "I" passes through on its path to earthly incarnation—the Moon sphere—it is appropriate that the corresponding fairy tale come at the conclusion of our study.

Some Characteristic Aspects of Silver

Silver has a unique relationship to light. Polished, the unalloyed metal has a brilliant luster and reflects objects more faithfully than any other metal. In combination with halogens it has the ability to preserve light impressions, thus laying the basis for photography—the creation of images of reality. Yet the reality it captures is only an instant that immediately becomes past; it plucks out of time single moments and fixes them in image form. One might say that the gift of silver is to make the present timeless—to reproduce the visible, material world and copy it ad infinitum.

When we look for corresponding processes in the human being, we find them in the regeneration and reproduction of cells in our organism; and these too have their basis in the Silver process. The principle at work in reproduction is heredity, the tendency of which is to bring forth the same type in endless repetition. As a physical phenomenon, human beings live on in this stream of heredity, by which the past is preserved in the descendents. In the life of the organism, on the other hand, the Silver dynamic is active in the anabolic (formative) forces.

---

1   Source: pitt.edu/~dash/ashliman.html. Translation: gutenberg2000.de /grimm/maerchen/6schwaen.html (revised).

Every organism needs to go through regular phases of regeneration to counteract the effects of fatigue and recoup exhausted forces—in other words, to restore freshness and vitality. It is the Silver process that enables us, in sleep, to perceive the spiritual archetype of our being as it was born out of the cosmos and to recreate ourselves in its image, in this way continually regenerating our organism. Connected with this is the elimination of substances no longer suitable for use in regeneration (excretion). The Silver process also has a cosmic regenerative aspect, which (in Selawry's interpretation) is portrayed in the Ariel scene at the beginning of part 2 in Goethe's *Faust*.[2]

The Motifs and Mood of the Tale
in relation to the Silver Process

The mood of this tale is set by the devotion and self-sacrifice of the sister toward her six enchanted brothers. In her quest to redeem them, no sacrifice is too great for her—not even that of her own life. The reader will recall a similar motif in "Faithful John," where we found the Lead process—the polar process to Silver—depicted. Because he may not speak, Faithful John is unable to defend himself against unjust accusations. Like him, the faithful sister here is unable to speak and prove her innocence; hence both are condemned to death. What gives them the capacity for sacrifice is loyalty: in the case of Faithful John, a servant's loyalty, which embodies the principle of selfless fulfillment of one's mission; and in the case of the sister, sisterly loyalty, embodying the principle of selfless devotion to others. This difference in motivation also illuminates a divergence on the soul level of these two figures. The soul gesture of the sister bears lunar character traits connected with the Silver process, which bestow the capacity for loving care of one's fellow man. This is a special capacity, found in certain individuals who feel particularly close to nature and love everything that is beautiful and harmonious. They have the gift of making everything around them grow and prosper. They will devote

---

2   Selawry, *Metallfunktionstypen in Psychologie und Medizin.*

themselves utterly to the wellbeing of those in their care; yet toward those who are not close friends or relatives, their attitude may be objective and distant, even critical, particularly if such people do not fit into their view of the world. This is the reverse side of the caring and nurturing quality we have described; yet it, too, stands under the soul aspect of the Moon sphere. Thus the behavior of the sister in "The Six Swans" provides us with a way of describing and studying the Silver process in its psychological and organic action.

Another central motif of this tale is the sister's silence; to fulfill the conditions for redeeming her brothers, she may not speak or laugh for six years and must sew six shirts from asters ("star flowers"). We will look further into the implications of her silence when we examine the specific images in the tale, but one aspect bears comment here. In the image of a sister stubbornly holding her silence and working at her sewing year after year, we recognize the musing soul, the dreamer who applies her imaginative powers to everything that touches her. The faculty of imagination—through which both outer impressions and inner prompting of the soul arise in our consciousness as images—is based on the Silver process. This central motif of this tale helps us characterize the Silver process, which is our aim in the following.

Moon Motifs

The fairy tale begins with the image of a king who has lost his way in the woods while out hunting. The "wild hunt" and "lost in the woods" are common fairy-tale motifs. In the picture language of the fairy tale, they generally signify an unrestrained instinctual life and sexual urge. As Drewermann has shown, the experience of the hunt has always been associated with virility and sexual conquest.[3] In this case they lead to a forced marriage. Thus what at first appears to be a random event becomes the logical consequence of thoughtless

---

3 Eugen Drewermann, "Lieb Schwesterlein, laß mich herein. Grimms Märchen tiefpsychologisch gedeutet," Munich, 1922, p. 420.

and unrestrained behavior. The union of the king with the witch's daughter, while forced and not consciously chosen, is at the same time a consequence of his "straying."

This introductory motif of the tale already brings us face to face with the mysterious and contradictory dynamic of Silver and the Moon. The Moon aspect of human life is the "night side of the soul," embracing everything that takes place unconsciously or semiconsciously in our soul life. Closely connected with this is our whole life of drives, including sexuality. The action of the Silver process in the organism begins with the genital organs. Even from a purely external point of view, the correspondence of the female monthly period to the twenty-eight-day lunar month testifies to the strength that these forces retain in the reproductive sphere.

The Past and the Silver Process

The Silver process, and the associated Moon sphere, is also the bearer and preserver of forces having to do with the past. Through the stream of heredity the Silver process forms the sheath into which the human soul-spirit enters at birth, thus allowing the past to act on into the present. Appropriately, then, the next motif in the fairy tale deals with the king's children. Even if he unwillingly agrees to a suspect marriage, the king still wishes to keep his children untouched by it—they are not to suffer from his "passion for hunting" or have anything to do with the new queen.

The tale draws particular attention to this aspect by telling of the king's previous marriage and his seven children from it—how he strives to keep his past secret from his second wife, how she discovers them and enchants the boys, and how thy fly away over the forest as swans.

The Moon Process and the External Sheaths of Life

How are these fairy-tale imaginations to be understood? Perhaps a word about the "stepmother" would be in order here—such a common motif in fairy tales and such an important, generally evil role.

Yet this very motif most clearly demonstrates that fairy-tale images never simply refer to everyday life. At the time when fairy tales arose and were collected, the stepmother was a common feature of families, since the biological mother so often died early in childbirth. Often the father had to remarry more than once to assure that all the tasks of keeping house and bringing up children could be properly done. Households tended to be large, especially when they were connected with a farm or craft workshop, and the mother's duties extended beyond the family to the employees.

It seems obvious that this is not the "stepmother" that we encounter in the fairy tales. In seeking another interpretation, we find a significant clue in the Latin word *mater* ("mother"), which is the origin of such words as *matter* and *materialism*. The lunar principle of *mater* has a wide scope, encompassing the entire aspect of creation that serves incarnation by connecting the spiritual being of man with earthly matter, thus forming our "material sheaths." In this sense the word "stepmother" (German *Stiefmutter*) can be understood as "stiff mother" (*"steife Mutter"*), the force that leads to densification in the material world, to connection with matter. The picture given by Rudolf Meyer is helpful here. "The whole material world in which we live eclipses the divine world today, so that we forget our spiritual home. In actual fact, materialism acts as a wicked stepmother, a stiff mother, toward our eternal being. The image is accurate."[4]

Returning now to our theme, we have seen that the Moon process enables the past to be "fixed." The stepmother in "The Six Swans" embodies this external aspect of the Silver process, whose nature it is to "enchant" everything it captures and at the same time to rob it of inner life. What is true of photography, in which the Silver process gives rise to an exact but lifeless image of reality, is also true of the stepmother's effect on the king's children. For the "six sons" are the sheaths that are acquired by the spirit-soul as it passes through the

---

4   Meyer, *The Wisdom of Fairy Tales.*

planetary spheres before reaching the lunar, the seventh sphere. It is these sheaths that the king wishes to preserve from enchantment.

The king (the "I") seeks to protect his children (or sheaths) from the influence of the stepmother (the Moon sphere). The fairy tale makes this clear through a series of striking images—the king leading his children to a secluded castle to hide them; their discovery by the stepmother (the soul-spirit cannot preserve its sheaths from the influence of the Moon sphere); the casting of charmed shirts over the six boys, robbing them of their human form; and their life in a feather-covered swan's body bereft of human inner life.

The swan has always been regarded as an image of the lunar element. The shimmering white coat of feathers is reminiscent of the pale light of the Moon. The long, slightly curving neck and small head give the bird an ethereal, dreamy appearance. The magical sight of a swan gliding peacefully on the water readily evokes the mood of a moonlit night.

The Silver Process and Imagination

Let us continue to interpret the rich imagery of this tale in terms of the Silver process. To release her brothers from their enchantment as swans, the princess must remain speechless for six years, nor may she laugh during this period. In addition, she must sew six shirts out of asters. What might it mean, to keep silent and not laugh? When the soul is held speechless, all of its inner stirrings are pent up. They cannot find utterance in language to communicate with the world; they cannot even find release in laughter. For when an impulse of the soul finds expression in language, it is put into conceptual form. While this represents a liberation, it is also a process of abstraction and fixation in which the original soul impulse loses its emotional intensity. It leaves the subjective realm of experience to be objectified in the sphere of language.

When the inner impulses of the soul cannot enter into outer life because speech and laughter are impossible, then they remain shut up within the soul and do not pass into conceptual formulation but into an image-based consciousness. In the soul there arises the fluid world of imagination. Imagination or pictorial consciousness is based on the Silver process and corresponds to the inner, psychic Moon aspect. The imaginative forces are connected with a process of interiorization, an enhancement of the inner powers. Through imagination, the soul can harbor longings and wishes and can learn to come to terms with them inwardly. Through the power of imagination, both joys and fears can be processed in a living way within the soul. In this way the human being grows in inner maturity and individual power.

This is the living process by which the human individuality gains strength; and this is why the healthy development of the imagination is of such importance for the child, who still must develop this individuality. Through it the child is able to take in the countless assailing foreign influences and transform them in a living way in a personal inner world. Imagination calls forth counter-images in the soul to the impressions of the outer world, neutralizing and overcoming them. This creates the free space necessary for the development of the individuality.

It is the Moon, or Silver process, that enables the soul to live out its impulses on the imaginative level. As we have indicated, the Silver process is one of reflection, which makes possible the image. In the soul these forces give rise to imaginative pictures. It is this process that is portrayed by the sister in the tale of "The Six Swans." She lives utterly in the forces of imagination, the picture world of her soul; no intellectuality, no conceptual thought expressed in language, is available to her. But through the power of imagination her individuality gains strength. We see this strengthening in the image of the heroine working tirelessly at sewing the six shirts out of asters, "star flowers." When the individuality develops, star forces can draw into it.

Strange as it may seem, the tasks performed by the imaginative forces in the soul realm are assumed in the bodily realm by the forces of inflammation. Just as the imagination resists external impressions that enter the soul, so the inflammatory process resists foreign substances that penetrate the organism.

The Formation of the Ether Body in the Moon Sphere

The image of shirts fashioned from "star flowers" has yet another significant aspect. When the human spirit being has arrived at the lunar sphere on its path toward incarnation from cosmic expanses, it now draws together its etheric or life body, the vehicle of its future life forces.[5] These forces depend on what the human entities living in the Moon sphere perceive as they contemplate the planets. In this light the "star shirts" can also be taken as a wonderful image for the etheric body as it is formed by the spirit body[6] in the lunar sphere on its path to Earth.

The Silver Process and the Continuity of Life

What if the Silver process is not controlled, however? Psychological stress cannot be properly processed in imaginative experience. The imagination slips off track because the soul is unwilling to accept being a mere mirror image, but wants to be in the center of the action. Feelings of rebellion, envy and desire arise in the soul. In the esoteric tradition such impulses, which also have a relation to the Moon process, were often connected with the image of the dragon. Thus in one of its meanings, the "dragon" is a soul impulse that would take everything into its possession, "swallowing up" human beings and taking total possession of them. The image of the demonic witch is fitting here; in fact, this case calls to mind King Macbeth and the three witches. The dragon is also a symbol of the forces that bring about the death of individual life. In many fairy tales and legends this theme is depicted in the image of the dragon who demands a human sacrifice as tribute—usually a king's daughter or son. The royal children may be taken as an image for the stream of heredity in its noblest form,

---

5   Steiner, *The Human Soul in Relation to World Evolution*, May 26, 1922, Dornach.

6   Sometimes also called *spirit man* (ed).

where it becomes most individualized and self-aware; this is what the forces of the dragon are intent on interrupting or destroying.

In the tale of "The Six Swans" this power appears in modified form. Here the false mother-in-law accuses the young queen of devouring her own children, insinuating that the young mother herself is an embodiment of these dragon forces. But the children are not dead! The wicked mother-in-law has stolen them away and hidden them, thus withholding them from their parents, but she has not dared to kill them. And since in fairy tales nothing is accidental, this detail too must have an exact meaning. In terms of the Silver process it implies that the stream of heredity can indeed be wrested away from the truly human level, even if it cannot be broken off.

If the demonic forces of the Moon had their way, it would continue only outwardly, unable to unite with the forces of human individualization. The children would not develop into true human beings—king's children—but stagnate on the purely biological level.

There is still another way of looking at this "kidnapping." Because the young queen has not yet reached the stage in her development where she is able to breathe individualized life into her sheaths ("release her brothers from enchantment"), the true being of her own children must remain foreign and hidden from her. As the reader will recall, the motif of children living in concealment was introduced at the beginning of the fairy tale. In both cases, despite their differences, the issue was keeping the children away from certain influences. And children always signify the future.

The Silver Process and Fever

The death sentence is to be carried out on the very day when the sister's six years of silence are completed. It is not coincidental that the death is to be by fire, for fire can be taken as an image for fever.

Fever is connected with an uncontrolled Silver process. The relationship between silver and fever is confirmed therapeutically, as *Argentum* in high potency is a well-proven remedy for debilitating fevers. Let us examine the process. In an attack of fever, the higher members of the human being—the "I" and astral body—engage directly in the physical body, bypassing the etheric body. Therefore they provoke a fever which literally "consumes" or "burns up" the organism. The effect of a focused silver therapy is to strengthen the etheric body in such a way that it is able to regain control of the anabolic processes and create a counterweight to the fever process. Under the influence of silver, the forces of the physical-etheric organization consolidate themselves.

It is important to know that fever is essentially imagination sunken to the biological level. In imagination it is the soul that becomes inflamed; in fever it is the body. The imaginative forces have shifted to the physical organism.

When we read that the young queen is to be burnt after six years of silence, we interpret this as indicating that the imaginative forces have become so intense that they threaten to move to the bodily nature. But this means that the moment has also arrived when the individuality can take hold of the Moon sheath and transform it. The shirts that the sister throws over the descending swans are the sheaths, now purified and imbued with star forces, in which the human soul-spirit will now be able to live; the brothers regain their human form. Only the youngest of them retains a swan wing, as his shirt is not quite finished. This youngest brother can be interpreted as representing the Mercury sphere, the last sphere through which the soul-spirit passes before entering the lunar sphere. Mercury was always depicted as having wings, and as the winged messenger of the gods he mediates between gods and humankind. Is this single wing that still remains on the youngest brother an indication that the human being, having become earthly, can still retain a connection, no matter how imperfect, to the divine world of spirit? We find justification for this view in the visual arts, where the degree of closeness to God was always expressed in the number of wings. Thus, the angels closest to God—the Seraphim—have six wings.

When the sister may finally speak again, she can expose the crimes of the mother-in-law, who is then burnt in her place. In other words, the derailed, uncontrolled Silver process, the "mother-in-law," now really leads to the acute phase of the fever, to "death by fire," which consumes the organism. Here the Silver process is corrupted with dragon power; it is no longer guided by moral force but by total self-absorption, which seizes the physical body. The body slips away from the soul and is seized by inflammatory processes. In this febrile storm the organism totally closes itself off from the outer world and consumes itself in an inner combustion process.

The Three Disease Tendencies in Connection with the Silver Process

Pursuing our medical considerations further and examining the entire fairy tale more closely, we find that certain images can be connected with an insufficiently strong Silver process and others to an overly strong one. The fairy-tale images not only enable us to recognize these disease pictures of a disturbed Silver process, but at the same time point toward ways of healing them.

The essential aspects of the Silver process are best illustrated by the example of the mirror. The mirror renders a clear image of reality, and the silver mirror does this most perfectly. No other mirror provides such a pure image; all other mirrors—the copper mirror—bring their own color to the image. It should be added that the mirror we picture here should not be a flat pane, but broken up, so that the image can go through multiple reduplications.

Thus the pure, selfless quality of the mirror makes possible a faithful image of reality; and a mirror image that can reflect itself gives rise to an endless repetition of that image. This can be taken as an image of the reproductive power of the Silver process. The forces of the Silver process act in the reproductive organs and so preserve the stream of heredity. The endless repetition of the same that is manifested in heredity is the mirror aspect of the Silver process. As mentioned, these forces of the Silver process can also be discovered in cell division and thus also in growth. From a spatial perspective the mirror represents a boundary that separates the mirror-space from the space outside. In this way there arises a space apart, which is delimited by a sheath, the mirror. This aspect points toward certain connections of the Silver process to the skin, in particular to the mucous membranes, the "boundary organ of the human organism."

In summary we may say that the Silver process manifests its nature on three planes, each of which can also be illustrated by the phenomena of the silver mirror. First, just as the mirror refuses to let an image pass through but casts it back, in imagination the impressions from the outer world are captured and processed as if on a picture screen. Second, as the mirror can produce unlimited copies of reality, in human reproduction the archetype of the body reappears in every child. Finally, just as the mirror is able simultaneously to delimit and to expand space, in the same way the skin and mucosae both delimit the organism from and expose it to the world without.

The Silver process can be disturbed in three directions. First, the inner mirroring can be too weakly developed, so that there is no clear imaginative awareness but only a dull state comparable to dream consciousness, and in some cases only a conceptual consciousness. Second, the delimiting function can be ineffective, giving rise to mucosal inflammations; or it can be excessive, so that the organism as a whole is isolated from the outer world, as occurs in a fever. Third, the forces of reproduction can be disturbed, giving rise to more or less severe pathologies of the reproductive organs.

Let us consider the fairy tale once more from this point of view. In the noble nature of the sister we see a properly developing Silver process. The stepmother and mother-in-law illustrate the Silver process that has slipped out of control and is pathologically exaggerated. The six swans, finally, offer the image of an overly weak Silver process.

In the sister, first, we see the particular human type who manifests a strong and harmonious Silver process. One embodiment of the healthy Silver process is a female figure—the self-sacrificing mother, the faithful sister, the devoted caregiver. As mentioned above, such a person has a special feeling for nature and its needs. She is concerned primarily with what lies close at hand and tends to the health and physical well-being of those entrusted to her care without tiring from the daily repetition. She finds fulfillment in providing loving care for family and those in her life community, and in creating a nourishing and cheerful environment for them. She is capable of great sacrifices to this end. Yet the powerfully developed Silver process also finds embodiment in quite another human type; the one for whom the development of the imagination becomes his profession, the creative artist. This is especially true of the author, the storyteller.

In our fairy tale it is sisterly love that stands in the foreground. For the sister, the redemption of her brothers is her heartfelt concern—her life's mission in fact. Therefore she never wavers, not even when surrounded by malicious suspicion, not even when threatened with the loss of her own life.

For this kind of sisterly love, freely chosen service to one's own takes precedence over everything else. The "domestic duties" (sewing the star-shirts) are tirelessly fulfilled day after day, testimony to an unquestioning devotion to those near and dear. As mentioned, another typical trait of the Silver type is a pronounced imagination. A rich soul life, formed and cultivated through inner discipline—six years of silence and six years without laughter—develops creative forces, which are the true "children of the spirit." This seems to be the meaning of the three children who, though at first withheld from the young queen, cannot really be taken from her. In the end she has everything; her royal spouse, her beautiful children and her redeemed brothers— the healthy "Silver person" is rich in beautiful human relationships.

Shock

Now we turn to the two deviations, keeping in mind the corresponding disease pictures. First, the weak Silver process is represented in the fairy tale by the transformation of the six brothers into swans. As we recall, this happens when white silk shirts containing an evil spell are cast over them. The white coat of feathers, the long neck, and the small head are an image of incomplete presence on the Earth. This transformation we interpret as an imaginative picture of shock. The spirit-being is shocked out of the body, lifted out of the earthly realm, so to speak. The weaker the Silver process—the less it fulfills its delimiting and enclosing functions—the more easily shock can set in. In such cases the Silver process can be strengthened therapeutically with low potencies of *Argentum* (for example, D6), which counteract the tendency to shock.[7] In the aftermath of a shock (and sometimes in other circumstances), individuals with a weak Silver process frequently have the sensation that their head is expanding, usually before falling asleep. This experience is based on an abnormal expansion of the etheric body beyond the bounds of the physical head, and thus is it quite rightly experienced as expansion. Here as well *Argentum* D6 is the indicated remedy. In cases of constitutional microcephaly (which an experienced physician can diagnose in early childhood), an extended "cure" of *Argentum* D6 may be indicated.

The image of the noiselessly gliding swan reminds us of yet another disease picture, sleepwalking. For the tendency to somnambulism, *Argentum* D6 again is the remedy of choice, as it strengthens the deficient boundary function of the Silver process.

Inflammation and Fever

The opposite picture—that of the over-powerful, uncontrolled Silver process—is portrayed by the stepmother and the mother-in-law. These two female figures realistically personify the self-absorbed, isolating Silver process. When the Silver process sinks too far into earthliness, the organism refuses to accommodate to the surrounding world and isolates itself completely. Thus, if we presently

---

7   Steiner, *Physiologisch-Therapeutisches auf Grundlage der Geisteswissenschaft* (Physiology and Therapeutics), Jan. 1, 1924, Dornach.

see inflammations—genuine febrile states—gaining in significance, it is a sign that forces of an "antisocial character," defensive forces proper, are at work. Fever is always an expression of an organism that is defending itself against what comes from without. In the process it can lose equilibrium and begin to consume itself. Then the organism loses the sense of living within the greater cosmic order and centers entirely on itself as the focal point of importance.[8] The therapy in these cases consists of *Argentum* in high potencies.

Illnesses of the Reproductive Organs

This revolt against all higher order can also play itself out on the plane of heredity. An excessive Silver process also tends to mount resistance to the stream of heredity because of the higher cosmic principle that lives in it.[9] Thus the genetic material, which is intended to work from the past through the present into the future, can be prevented by certain ailments from fulfilling its immediate tasks (the brothers are enchanted into swans). A second aspect of this revolt, an intensification of the first, is the attempt to actually interrupt the stream of heredity. As we have already shown, this process occurring in the depths of the organism can be pictured in the image of the dragon, the "eater of humans," intent on usurping the high cosmic order of reproduction. Clinical disease pictures corresponding to an uncontrolled, excessive Silver process are conception disorders, sterility, inflammations of the reproductive organs, amenorrhoe, etc. Treatment consists of *Argentum* preparations in injection form at potencies from D20 to D30.

Cancer and the Imagination

There is one further pathology that properly belongs to this discussion, although we find no direct correspondence to it in the tale of "The Six Swans." Nevertheless, a connection exists that enables

---

8   Steiner, *True and False Paths in Spiritual Investigation*, Aug. 15, 1924, Torquay, UK.

9   Ibid.

us to cast light on certain therapeutic aspects. We are speaking of the disease of cancer, in particular solid cancer in adults. Cancer is characterized by unbridled cell division and cell growth that the organism is unable to control. On the cellular level it is an endless "reproduction of the same" that gives rise to the tumor; and in this dynamic, too, we recognize one aspect of a degenerated Silver process. Yet there are also other aspects of the Silver process that develop in an uncontrolled manner in cancer. Cancer patients can be described as becoming altogether "Moon-like," losing all light and inner luminosity of their own. It is as though, like the Moon, they are only able to reflect outer light. In anthroposophic medicine cancer is treated with mistletoe, which can be called a "Moon plant" because it retains a direct connection to the "old Moon" and reflects conditions that reigned in that age.

Certain forms of psychotherapy used as adjunctive cancer treatment (and developed independently from Spiritual Science) can also be related to the Moon process.[10] The best known of these is the visualization or imagination technique of American physician Simonton. In his approach, cancer patients learn to apply their will to the imagination. They visualize the cancer, picturing the cancer cells as dragons seeking to destroy their body and their own cells as knights heroically battling the dragons and seeking to kill them. The use of such mental imagery enables patients to confront their illness.[11]

Pictures have a completely different meaning for the soul than concepts. Pictures offer a projection field that enables the soul to identify with them. Pictures completely take hold of the soul, and in learning to produce them patients necessarily develop a power that

---

10   J. Barthoweak et al., "Imaginationen und Gruppentherapie: ein neues Behandlungsprogramm zur Bewältigung der Krebsnachsorge," *Krebsgeschehen* 2, 1986.

11   Such visualization techniques are based on a different image of the human being than that of our study. The resulting issues and limitations are discussed by R. F. Wagner in his study "Psychologische Intervention in der Krebstherapie. Gedanken zu einem sogenannten ganzheitlichen Modell der Kreibsheilung," *Beiträge zu einer Erweiterung der Heilkunst* 1, 1983.

guides their own inner impulses and develops their moral imagination. Pictures evoke a living experience of evil and good that challenges the human being to come to terms with them.

The same cannot be said of abstractions. When soul impulses are formulated conceptually, they pass through an abstraction process that leaves only that which is exactly defined and fixed. This cannot set our moral forces afire and therefore hardly makes an impression on the inmost soul. The abstraction process externalizes the impulses of the soul, so that they fail to penetrate to the deepest layers. When abstraction becomes the dominant or exclusive mode of the soul, then those forces within it that ought to develop "soul backbone" and strengthen the individuality are left unawakened. These forces not awakened by imagination then sink to the bodily level, and what should have been actualized in the soul realm now plays itself out in the organic sphere. Figuratively speaking, untransformed dragon forces in the soul now take hold of the cells and lead to uncontrolled growth. A confrontation takes place on the organic level that properly should have been met by the soul in an earlier phase of life. This displacement to a different level was necessary because the undeveloped imagination was unable to battle the dragon in the soul.

Simonton's visualization technique and other imaginatively based approaches can be understood as attempts to draw the sunken forces now slumbering on the physical level back up to the soul level. These patients need to make up for a process that they failed to go through earlier, perhaps due to an emphasis on abstract intellectual thinking in childhood and adolescence.[12] They must learn belatedly to develop their imaginative faculty. Essentially they are going through the process that the sister in "The Six Swans" had pass through in her six years of suffering. Just as the development of imagination guides

---

12 Michael Holm-Hadulla determined in his investigations that cancer patients characteristically display limited imaginative activity. Hence, they are unable to experience psychological problems symbolically or pictorially or to process them on this plane (Holm-Hadulla, *Psychologische Aspekte der Krebskerkrankung*).

the silver process in the fairy tale and leads to redemption from the "Moon world," so the training of the imagination offers the cancer patient help in combating the "Moon illness" of cancer.

It is astonishing how the various aspects we have found connected with the Moon process fit together to produce a well-rounded picture. In spite of their colorful variety, like mosaic pieces joined together correctly they unite to create a clear picture. The virtue of a synthetic view of the fairy tale and therapy is that it offers a better understanding of the particular form of therapy while at the same time confirming the truth content of the fairy tale.

FAIRY TALES AND UNDERSTANDING THE METALLIC REMEDIES

Interpreting Fairy Tales: Methodology and Reliability

Has this study exhausted all the interpretative possibilities of the fairy tales it has examined?[1] Far from it! Fairy tales, like life itself, are an inexhaustible source of fresh insight and knowledge, and the vast literature on the subject clearly shows how variously they can be experienced and interpreted. They speak differently to each of us, and we each interpret them according to our own sensibility and faculties. Yet the contradictions between different ways of understanding the fairy tales are for the most part only apparent and are often resolved when the differences in point of view are recognized. The present investigation represents but one of numerous possible approaches to the world of the fairy tale.

That having been said, this study does possess one feature that distinguishes it from a great many others. Its conclusions have always been confirmed in practical medical experience with remedies. This has made it possible not only to cast a fresh light on the fairy tales but also to develop a new understanding of the metal remedies. Numerous therapeutic experiences with the metal remedies can now be viewed in a context out of which new treatments can be derived. Particular fairy tales open up better access, or even entirely new access, to knowledge of the spiritual interrelatedness of metal remedies, planetary forces, and the human being—knowledge that enables the physician in a spiritually extended medical practice to explore new avenues in metal therapy and to apply them in a wide

---

1   This conclusion refers in part to the chapter on Character Typology, which is not included in this translation (TN).

variety of illnesses. In such cases the relationship between fairy tale and remedy finds practical therapeutic confirmation in a striking way.

Our investigation has resulted in a remarkable insight, namely that the "message" of the fairy tales—what they wish to communicate through their image-language—is actually embodied in the very substance of the remedies we have studied here. Concealed within the fairy tales is knowledge of the spiritual healing forces at work in the human being; for that reason, they can reveal to our understanding the remedies' mode of efficacy. Metal as remedy and human being as patient are a match for one another—they are related because in the ideal sphere they form a unity. The study of fairy tales makes a significant contribution to understanding this unity. In particular, it makes obvious that the curative action of these preparations cannot be of a material nature—that is, it must take place entirely on the spiritual plane.

Such evidence, based as it is on medical experience and remedy provings, may not offer proof in the conventional scientific sense; yet it is so extensive, and some of it so thoroughly documented through a range of therapeutic approaches (homeopathy and anthroposophic medicine among them), that it cannot simply be dismissed as speculative. Furthermore, anyone willing to look into this evidence will be able to recognize the connections on a cognitive level and so gain an inner relationship to them.

It is characteristic of our response to such insights—as to any fairy-tale interpretations—that we accept or reject them according to our personal sense of truth. Whether they are of interest and significance to us, or whether we are even able to receive them without pre-judgment, is entirely a matter of our own convictions.

In natural science this freedom does not exist. "Unambiguous evidence" forces us to accept certain conclusions. In addition, scientifically proven results inevitably lead to practical technological applications, where their correctness can no longer be doubted. In medicine, too, the particular triumphs of the scientific method have been in the area where it plays the most crucial role—the high-tech sphere. Here, no space exists for questions about the true nature or meaning of illness. Thus, the proofs of natural science possess validity only in the sphere to which they apply—the technical side of the world—but not in the area containing the spiritual side of the human being and the world. Ultimately, then, these proofs and results remain one-sided. The world of life and spirit, the world that is captured in fairy tales, eludes proof in this form; it can be recognized only in freedom and out of loving engagement. As an observer one must sense the truth oneself; and the "proof" in such cases comes about through devotion, interest, perception, understanding, and one's own attitude toward life.

It is from this perspective that the results of this study should be received. Its particular concern is to include spiritual aspects in our understanding of remedies. Method plays a central role here; hence the emphasis of this study falls on describing the path of imaginative research and highlighting its categorical difference from the methods of natural science. The intent is to show that the inward path— meditative experience of an inner, spiritual world—can also yield objective knowledge with practical consequences for therapies and the manufacture of remedies.

This approach unites the artistic—the element of the fairy tale— with the scientific—the basis for understanding the action of remedies. The artistic is an individual approach that involves the entire human being. Its starting point is the individual's capacities for experiencing. The scientific, in contrast, is based on our intellectual powers and is limited to the head forces. Out of the union of these two approaches a method is born that we might call artistic science or science of the living. This is the method suited to understanding the remedies under consideration here.

Although this approach is not new, we still stand at its beginning as a method of research. If it is to gain importance, it requires significant extension and deepening. In particular, if we as specialists and laypersons wish to overcome our largely unintentional and frequently unconscious habits of thought regarding health, sickness, and healing, then our approach needs to meet with more general interest and understanding. Only through an artistic science can we reach a new understanding of diseases and remedies.

The Unity of Humanity and Nature, Disease, and Illness

From the special perspective of the fairy tales we have been able to reveal connections—doubtless unfamiliar ones to most readers—between humankind, metal, and the planetary sphere. Things that seem, from the earthly perspective, infinite in their variety and dispersion, such as the occurrence of metals and metal compounds in nature, prove from a cosmological-spiritual viewpoint to be related and interwoven. By working toward an understanding of the picture-language of fairy tales we have been able to practice this viewpoint, experiencing the metals not merely as dead substances, but as something whose essential nature is closely akin to our own spiritual nature as human beings.

Such knowledge of the spiritual nature of metals, which was inaccessible to our earthly senses, not only opens new avenues in therapy, it also opens our eyes to dangers to which all people are exposed in the course of their lives—biographical crises and disease tendencies. In the metals, we have been able to recognize natural images that bear an inner kinship to specific character structures of the human being. It turns out that on the spiritual path, knowledge of nature and man is always linked to knowledge of the self. The path of self-knowledge poses a definite challenge to each human being, for as a rule the area that we know least and where we are most exposed to deception is our own selves. Yet this is an essential condition for living a more conscious life.

Thus in their inner nature, the metals bear a close relationship to the inner development and maturation of the human being. This accounts for their centrality in anthroposophic medicine. Although the approach we have taken here is limited to the seven planetary metals, it can be seen as a model for spiritual contemplation of material substance altogether. In appropriate form it can also be applied to the plant and animal kingdoms as well. No matter where we turn our gaze in nature, we see more than an external given; we experience also a counterpart to ourselves. When we recognize this we will perceive natural substances in a new light and feel our kinship with them. We will be able to enter into an intimate dialogue with them. When we make use of their healing forces, instead of taking them for granted we will feel how indebted we are to the entire realm of nature. This is the sentiment expressed in Christian Morgenstern's poem "The Washing of the Feet":

> I thank you, silent stone of earth,
> and gently lean to you beneath.
> My life as plant I owe to you.

> I thank you, grounds and meadows green,
> and bend down close to you beneath.
> My life as animal depends on you.

> I thank you animal and plant and stone,
> and bow down thankfully to you beneath.
> You helped me to become, all three.

> We give you thanks, oh human child,
> And kneel in reverence before you;
> For because you are, we are.

> And thanks resound from all God's oneness
> And all God's manifoldness;
> In thanks all being intertwines.[2]

Anthroposophic Medicine as Mystery Medicine

Faced with the almost unfathomable scope of fairy-tale wisdom— the wisdom of human individuals, humanity, and the world—the reader may wonder how people could possibly have apprehended it

---

2   Christian Morgenstern, "Die Fußwaschung," Munich, 1959. Translation adapted from http://strayandfancy.blogspot.com/2010/11/advent.html.

and transformed it into fairy-tale images. As we explained in the introduction, in earlier times spiritual adepts and initiates were trained at certain mystery centers to perceive the action of the metal forces in the human being and in the world, and so had deep experiences characterized by inspirations. We must assume (as Rudolf Steiner indicates) that as part of this process they took in metallic compounds in high dilutions—high potencies, we would say today—and that due to the particular inner constitution of the adepts at the mystery centers at that time, their souls were able to experience images of the particular "wisdoms" connected with these substances. When these high dilutions were ingested, it was as though the planetary gods themselves spoke to the initiates and communicated cosmic thoughts to them in images. It is likely that it was also in this way the fairy-tale images first arose, which would explain their direct connection to particular substances. This would also make sense of the close connections between medicinal remedies and fairy-tale images. Just as homeopathic remedy pictures still reveal profound mysteries today, at that time adepts, with their particular soul constitution, were able on a much greater scale to experience insights of wisdom in the form of Imaginations by taking in high dilutions.

To better understand the world of the ancient mysteries, where "physician" and "priest" were the same, we must bear in mind that disease and health were experienced altogether differently than is the case today. The overarching experiences at that time were of harmony and disharmony with the cosmos, and these were experienced not as principles but as the activities of a multiplicity of divine agencies in humanity and the world. The initiates directed their vision toward the invisible world, the world of forces hidden behind the manifest world. This world of forces was experienced as divine and thus as enduring. The physician in the ancient mysteries acted from such knowledge of the spiritual connections between humankind and nature and experienced the self as a part of this spiritual world.

When we come to the time of Paracelsus,[3] we see humankind pictured as a little cosmos (microcosm) that corresponds to the great cosmos (macrocosm) of all creation.

Thus knowledge of the relationship described here between metals and humankind is not new. It is possible to trace—as we have just done—a direct thread running from the mystery centers of ancient Greece to anthroposophic medicine. The Eleusinian Mystery centers of ancient Greece cultivated knowledge and experiences of the connection of the metals to the spiritual nature of humanity and the planetary forces. A corresponding worldview is also found in Neoplatonism and in Gnosticism. In the Middle Ages this knowledge was developed further in a hermetic circle of the Rosicrucian stream. By them (among others) it was spread in disguised form—such as fairy tales—and so it was able to enter into the soul life of the common folk. In a new form this knowledge has been made accessible and comprehensible to our present-day consciousness through Rudolf Steiner's Spiritual Science. It becomes clear that anthroposophic medicine, at least in its knowledge of remedies, has developed out of ancient mystery knowledge; in this sense it is a further development of mystery wisdom in a contemporary form. With this connection, the spiritual background of this form of medicine is made perfectly clear.

In our day, the path leading to a spiritualized medicine requires not only acquiring professional skills but also taking personal responsibility for consciously schooling and developing the inner life. Only with these will our outward and inward perceptions lead to the kind of experiences that offer direct spiritual cognition of nature and the human being. Rudolf Steiner has set out in detail the paths that lead in this direction. One stage on this path entails exercises for Imaginative cognition, and our endeavor here has been to apply them to an in-depth examination of the fairy tales and so to demonstrate what sort of knowledge can result.

---

3   The years 1493 to 1541 (TN).

Fairy Tales and Alchemy

To readers who have experienced doubts and questions regarding our approach, the following section on the relationship of certain fairy tales to alchemical processes employed in anthroposophic pharmacy will likely make even less sense, because these processes are based on an understanding of substance and remedy that is diametrically opposed to the active-agent paradigm of conventional medicine and science today. At this point we also leave behind the domain of homeopathic remedy pictures, which provided a certain experimental validation and reliability to our findings. The following presentation may therefore appear speculative, and it will also have to remain quite aphoristic. Nevertheless it is worth presenting here because it brings out in a concrete manner the link between the Rosicrucian wisdom of those who created the fairy tales and the spiritual understanding of remedies in anthroposophic medicine.

The remedies in question here are preparations whose production bears a close relationship to Paracelsian manufacturing processes and can therefore be described as alchemical.

The connections between alchemy and fairy tales have been noted by a number of authors.[4] Let us first point to some of the general correspondences. The central focus of both fairy tales and alchemy is on processes of transformation. The point of the fairy tale is not that its characters gain experience, knowledge, or skills, but that they undergo a transformation. Let us call to mind a few of the fairy-tale motifs we have encountered in this book; the old servant John, stiffened in death, becomes a new John full of youthful vigor; a Goose Girl who is actually a princess becomes a queen; wild-man Iron Hans becomes a mighty king, as he was originally; Lucky (and naïve) Hans, repeatedly manipulated by his desires, appears in the end as a joyous person in harmony with himself; Snow White, pursued and living in hiding, become a queen as befits her high lineage; the enchanted swan-brothers regain their human form; and so on and so forth. The

---

4   For example, Roger, *A la découverte de l'alchimie*, pp. 77–231.

concern of the fairy tale is not that its hero will have more, or be more, at the end than at the beginning—in fact, fairy-tale heroes of royal origin frequently regain their royalty only through humiliation. The point is rather that they are transformed. Essentially they have everything already; they do not need to acquire additional things or qualities. Their destiny is to be completely "recast," no longer to be the same person they were at the beginning.

It is similar with the production of alchemical remedies; the primary concern is the transformation of substance, not its alteration, isolation or standardization in a chemical sense. And just as the plot of fairy tales seems to unfold on a plane outside of ordinary reality, so the alchemical process seems to bear no relation to the physio-chemical laws of the earthly world. And yet not randomness, but a strict inner lawfulness holds sway both in the fairy tale and in alchemy. The discussion of our seven chosen fairy tales has revealed the high nature of these laws, which derive from the spiritual plane and embody both past and future aspects of the cosmos and humanity.

In this sense alchemy is a concealed philosophy of spiritual development and evolution—that is, an approach toward the development of the individual, humanity, and the world from a spiritual perspective. On a small scale—using substances in a laboratory retort—alchemy reenacts the cosmic creation process of the past and enacts the redemptive work of the future. If this claim appears speculative, senseless, or perhaps even arrogant to modern eyes, let the reader consider where science is going in the field of gene technology. Is it not pursuing comparable goals, even if on a completely different—profane—level? Alchemy understands its intention as the perfection of nature from the point of view of a spiritual cosmogony and accords a crucial role to revealed knowledge, while gene technology sees itself as "correcting" or "improving" creation from a profane material perspective guided by the researcher's own intellectual powers.

Forces that guide the upward development, transformation and redemption of the world and humanity—forces of which the alchemy of Paracelsus and others cultivated a practical knowledge—appear either as illusory or magical to the profane worldview. From a spiritual point of view these are wisdom-filled creation-forces, cosmic intelligences whose agency is called into play in the transformative alchemical process. Use of these forces is guided by a hidden ethic that stands in harmony with the spiritual laws of the world's development.

Thus alchemical practice revolves around cosmogonic models as transformational motifs for humankind and matter. This is the aspect of it that is truly creative, the aspect that extends far beyond the laboratory and beyond accepted concepts of matter. However, if one wishes to understand the alchemical art one needs to understand these cosmogonic laws—laws which are at work in the human being, too, of course.

An example will help to clarify the alchemical perspective. For the production of certain remedies, Rudolf Steiner indicates that the metals we have examined in this book must undergo a profound transformation—Steiner calls it "re-casting" (*Umformung*). First they are subjected to a variety of dissolving processes using acids and heating, then to combining processes involving precipitation and drawing off, thus bringing them into a perfected, non-metallic form. In the next step, suitable plants are fertilized with these transformed metals. In the resulting intimate union with the plant, the metal is raised to a higher level, etherized, and restored to inner kinship with the light. It has been released from its earthly form and transformed into a light substance. This method gives rise to the preparations marketed by Weleda as "vegetabilized metals."

From the chemical point of view, it is impossible to detect an elevated metal content in plants so fertilized, and this fact might seem to invalidate the whole procedure as a pharmaceutical concept. Yet the plant itself displays an altered appearance, a more intense green for example, from which we conclude that it has united itself more strongly with the light.

In this production process the metals are divested of their specifically metallic properties. Released from their earthbound condition, they can rise wholly into the plant's light realm. And through this transformation and elevation, the essential being of the metal finds it way back to its true origin—what the language of the fairy tale would call its kingly lineage; for originally, before they took on material form as earthly elements, the metals were "servants and kinfolk" of the light. Through the production process of vegetabilized metals, they are released from their earthly bondage—from material enchantment—to regain the realm of light.

"Hans in Luck" offers some striking parallels to the process we are describing. A metal used in the production of vegetabilized metal remedies—a lump of gold—sets the action in motion and plays a central role throughout the story. Through a bizarre series of adventures, this gold is progressively stripped of its earthly value. Yet far from becoming worthless, in a spiritual sense it casts its light over the entire development by which Hans ultimately becomes a "Sun child." "There is no man under the Sun so fortunate as I," he exclaims at the end of the tale, when his gold has lost the last vestige of its earthly value and sunk to the bottom of the well in the form of a common whetstone.

What is carried out externally as a pharmaceutical process in the production of the vegetabilized metals appears in a totally different form in the fairy tale, where it is depicted in images that enable us to experience the transformation of external gold into an inner quality. The two sets of steps—that of the fairy tale and that of the pharmaceutical process—correspond to one another. The external, sense-perceptible alchemical process that leads to the remedy is echoed by an inner process within the human being, who is likewise an image of the great cosmic creative process. These different perspectives on the same course of events are characteristic of the Paracelsian alchemical worldview. The fairy tale allows us to experience the inner development, and this can help us to understand the outward alchemical procedure.

With all of these considerations we have not even touched on the therapeutic value of these preparations. But this is a topic that goes beyond the scope of this study and must be left to another occasion. We shall only point out that the remedies produced in this manner are particularly effective on the nerve-sense system.

Let us consider one more example, this one showing the transformation of metallic lead into a remedy that can address geriatric illnesses and lead to a kind of spiritual rejuvenation. The manufacture of this preparation too is based on indications by Rudolf Steiner and occurs as follows: lead is melted, poured into a honeycomb mold, and the resulting cast filled with honey. The honey-filled lead cast is then ground up, melted, and again made into honeycomb mold, which this time is filled with sugar. This preparation, too, is ground and then potentized to a high potency, at which point it is ready for use as a remedy.

From the chemical point of view this procedure must appear incomprehensible. If it were not possible to demonstrate its clear efficacy in geriatric illnesses, the entire idea would have to be dismissed as nonsense. However, the lead tale of "Faithful John" offers us help in our attempt to understand the composition of the preparation by revealing the cosmogonic principles on which it is modeled.

In our discussion of the tale of "Faithful John," we pointed out that it is a depiction of cosmogony, that is, of aspects of human and cosmic development in the widest possible sense. From an imaginative perspective it reflects three such phases—the condition of ancient Saturn, the preceding state of cosmic oneness with the light (to Jakob Böhme, the harmony of all creation through the divine Sophia), and the re-attainment of this condition for a future humanity. The reunion with the forces of light is represented by the union of the King with Princess of the Golden Dome. And in a mysterious way both the death and the rejuvenation of faithful servant John are bound up with this process. In our interpretation, the image of the Princess of the Golden Dome represents the divine forces of wisdom and love.[5]

---

5   This was pointed out earlier by Arthur Schult and Rudolf Meyer. For discussion, please refer to the section on the relevant fairy tale in this book.

When we look at the lead-honey-sugar preparation from the cosmogonic viewpoint, we can see these substances as representatives of particular steps in the development and transformation of the individual and of humanity as a whole. In the case of lead, we found that it has preserved forces of the ancient Saturn condition. Since to apply this approach thoroughly to both honey and sugar would go beyond the scope of this chapter, we shall limit ourselves to honey here. Honey is a light substance. We can begin to understand this statement by looking at honey in the context of bee nature. In all of its activities, the bee is oriented entirely toward the light of the Sun. Lorenzen[6] makes a convincing case that as a spiritual entity, the bees did not participate in the great fall in which primal humanity fell from light-filled cosmic harmony, and so in a certain way they have preserved the preceding condition. Thus in honey we have a substance that comes into being out of a Sun-oriented activity that the bees have carried over from the pre-Saturn world. If the Saturn process can be described as a condition of darkness resulting from the loss of the divine light, then honey embodies the polar condition: intimate kinship with light. From this perspective we can look on honey as the earthly representative of the cosmic forces—or beings—of light and wisdom which Jakob Böhme spoke of as the Divine Sophia. And if we acknowledge this as the essential dynamic of honey, we may also surmise that Rudolf Steiner saw honey as a polarity to lead and thus as a force helping to prevent humanity falling back into the "Saturn condition."

Mediating between the forces of lead and honey is sugar; it might be called the "binding agent" that enables the polarities to come into connection with one another. However, it is not possible to go further into this here.

Thus we see that what originally formed a unity in human and cosmic evolution and then fell apart—as discussed in the chapter on "Faithful John"—is alchemically reunited here with "cosmogonic" forces on the plane of substance. Thus this preparation actually

---

6   Lorenzen, *Metamorphosen*, Verlag für zeitgemäßen Goetheanismus.

contains within itself an evolutionary and transformational path that leads from ancient Saturn to the future stage when human evolution is to be reunited with the forces of light, the forces of fire. Steiner calls this future condition of Earth and human evolution the Venus condition.

The diseases of old age correspond to the Saturn condition; they are a relapse of the patient, as it were, to the ancient Saturn stage of evolution. As a force, honey contains the future condition that Steiner calls the Venus stage of evolution, and thus, when used rightly as a remedy, it helps overcome geriatric disease.

Our intention here has not been to go into the manufacture of alchemical remedies—hence the brevity of these indications—but only to point to certain relationships between alchemy and fairy tales that can help us better understand Steiner's remedy compositions.

Summary and Preview of Further Imaginative Remedy Studies

In these studies of fairy tales, we have shown that the seven metal processes stand in relation to seven corresponding organ formations, seven metabolic processes, seven soul dispositions, and seven virtues, and that they can be seen as paths of "inner maturation." We have spanned an arc from human beings to metal to planetary sphere; and in understanding this great arc, the fairy tales were of decisive help to us. Through their images we were able point out how particular organs, metabolic processes, functional activities, and soul-spiritual constitutions are linked to the metals. In this way we have recognized that the essential "being" of the metals is active on four different levels in our organism, and that metal preparations are effective as remedies for diseases in these areas.

Of these aspects, the relation of fairy-tale images to soul development and inner growth is particularly palpable; and this is why we have devoted particular attention to this aspect. Using the fairy tales, we have attempted to show how inner transformation and maturation are connected with planetary processes in the astral body, and we have found that this process can be divided into three phases, of which the last in particular must be consciously undertaken by the human "I." In the first two phases as well, the guidance and harmonizing action of the "I" are needed, but on these levels it is supported by the forces of the bodily organization and the model of the adults responsible for our growth and education.

As complex as it is, a discussion of the action of the metal processes in the human being fails to address all aspects of the human being. For beyond the planets, the zodiac has from time immemorial been seen as a formative influence on human beings. The human form in its totality has always been seen in connection with the action of zodiacal forces. Therapeutic experience has shown that remedies connected with the zodiac have a particular effect on our bodily constitution as well as on characteristics and capacities of the self—the way in which we become conscious of the world and develop a corresponding worldview and manner of behavior.

Emanating from the twelve directions the zodiac are the fundamental moods that are taken up in particular ways by the planets. Thus, depending on the zodiacal sign it stands in front of, the Sun mediates a different mood to the Earth and to human beings. This is true in a corresponding way of the other six planets as well. Thus it is not just a question of moving from seven-ness to the twelve of the zodiac; for there are actually seven times twelve different influences to reckon with—and more, if the interactions are considered in a more differentiated way.

We may assume that the initiates of earlier times ingested not only highly diluted metals but also non-metals, for example certain salts and plants, which stand in connection with the action of the zodiac. If so, then we may assume that the essential dynamic of these substances as well was grasped and has found expression in the image language of the fairy tales. Preliminary studies, not yet fully articulated or published, point in this direction.

In this book we have investigated seven of the two hundred total fairy tales in the Grimms' collection. It surely contains a number of tales dealing with various aspects of the zodiac, alone or in interaction with the planets. Using these fairy tales it should be possible to explore other remedies and diseases. In fact, it may well be possible to offer a similar discussion based on fairy-tale imaginations for the majority of the anthroposophic and homeopathic remedies.

From this point of view the present study represents only a beginning, one that may be well rounded thematically but has taken only a single step on the path toward a spiritual pharmacology that combines conceptual understanding with imaginative experience. Thus one can have an intimation of the immeasurable treasury of undisclosed truth and wisdom that remains ours to discover in the fairy tales. It also becomes clear that the anthroposophic and homeopathic remedies still harbor many undisclosed insights about the human being and about the relationships of the human being to the world.

Appendix: Therapeutic Applications of the Seven Planetary Metals

The following tables list remedy pictures for the seven planetary metals and their compounds. They give the abstract terms corresponding to the imaginative disease pictures that we have developed out of our work with the fairy tales. We saw the images in the fairy tales as imaginative, living remedy pictures. Because these retain the cosmological connection, they correspond to the essential anthroposophic understanding of remedies. The remedy pictures listed below, in contrast, relate only to pathological symptoms and make no overarching connections. Remedy pictures of this kind ignore aspects that are essential to an understanding of anthroposophic remedies.

These tables are based in large part on materials which the author, in the course of his professional life, has culled from the voluminous record of medical experience published in the anthroposophic medical literature. The tables are intended to provide the medically knowledgeable reader with an overview of the therapeutic uses of the metal remedies. The starting point in each table is the healthy condition, reflecting a balanced metal process. The middle column of the table begins with keywords describing this condition and then lists the character typology corresponding to each area of soul life.

To either side of this are listed pathological alterations and disorders—on the left, those that result from one-sided and/or excessive metal processes; on the right, those that result from deficient metal processes. Each disease listing is followed by the appropriate metal remedy, which is given in the customary potency. It will be noticed that high potencies are indicated for the excessive and one-sided metal processes, while low potencies are used for the insufficient metal processes.

The assignment of the individual diseases was based on external criteria, but it could easily be done differently.

Simplification facilitates an overview, and this is why the tables have been provided. As we have said, however, their schematic nature makes it necessary to neglect certain aspects. The aspects of time and functional threefold nature, for example, are not considered in the tables although they play an important role in the choice of potency. It is not always just the disease picture that is decisive in choosing the potency level; it also depends on the plane (in terms of functional threefold nature) on which we intend to address the disease process. Depending on whether we wish to address it from the metabolic area, from the rhythmic area or from the nerve-sense area, we will choose the potencies accordingly. High potencies act on the nerve-sense system, middle ones on the rhythmic processes, and low ones on the metabolic processes. The phase of a disease also plays a role in choosing potencies. In the acute phase lower potencies tend to be appropriate, while in the healing phase and for chronic illnesses, higher potencies will be preferred. Another possible factor in potency choice is the patient's temperament. A sanguine individual will respond better to high potencies, while the hypochondriac will more often require lower potencies. As the dynamic of the disease process also shifts over the human lifetime, younger patients are better treated with lower potencies, older ones with higher potencies. Additionally, the remedy itself plays an important role in the choice of potency.

Thus, quite a number of aspects are left out of consideration in the tables on the following pages.

Lead Remedies

Area of Efficacy and Therapeutic Applications

Excessive or one-sided lead processes and corresponding remedies	Balanced lead processes and functional areas	Weak, deficient lead processes and corresponding remedies
	Soul Area	
Immobile, abstract, egocentric in soul life,	"Melancholic" temperament	Underdeveloped and immature; poor psychological boundaries
Obstinate, resentful, opinionated, obsessive ideas (*Plumbum* D30);	Good memory, abstract thinking; principled, thorough; lives according to convictions; enthusiastic, inner fire; discriminating; self-contained; profound	No distance, infantility, addictions, alcoholism (*Minium* D4, D6);
Forgetful/distracted (*Scleron*);		Agitation (*Plumbum chloratum* D4 – D6)
Autistic spectrum (*Plumbum silicicum* D20);		
Isolated/depressed, incapable of enthusiasm, hypochondria (*Plumbum* D20);		
Perverse instincts (*Plumbum silicicum* D20);		
Dementia (*Plumbum* D30)		

Process and Organ Areas I.

Becomes too rigidly and firmly anchored in the self-space, destructive inner warmth	Forms a unified self-space, spatially consolidated and revitalized with inner warmth	Self-space is insufficiently delimited and protected, insufficient inner warmth
Thin physique, low energy with dry, wrinkly skin (*Plumbum* D14 – D30);		Obesity (*Plumbum* D6 – D8);
Allergies, autoaggressive diseases (*Plumbum* D14 – D20);		Epilespy (*Plumbum* D6);
Bleeding (*Plumbum* D30);		Cramps, colics (*Plumbum aceticum* D3 – D6);
Intermittent claudication, pale hypertension (*Plumbum mellitum* D20);		Chronic spastic constipation (*Plumbum* D10);
Cramps, epilepsy (*Plumbum* D20);		Chronic polyarthritis (*Plumbum* D6, *Cerussit* D6, *Galenit comp.*)
Hydrosis, aphonia, laryngospasm, childhood aphasia (*Plumbum* D30);		
Sleeplessness (*Plumbum* D20);		
Chronic nephritis, nephrosclerosis (*Galenit* D20)		

Process and Organ Areas II.

Excessive or displaced mineralization	Mineralization, ossification and hemopoiesis, dying process in space, warmth process in temporal bloodstream	Deficient mineralization
Arteriosclerosis, sclerosis (*Scleron, Plumbum mellitum* D20); Tinnitus (*Plumbum* D20); Macular degeneration (*Galenit* D20); Scleroderma (*Plumbum* D20, *Plumbum silicicum* D15); Osteoarthritis, spinal disc degeneration (*Plumbum silicicum* D15); Neuropathy (*Plumbum* D30)		Rickets, osteomalacia (*Galenit* D6, *Plumbum* D10); Arthritis, gout (*Galenit* D4); Obesity (*Plumbum* D6, D8); Weak ligaments, senile pruritis (*Plumbum silicicum* D10); Sensation disorders (*Plumbum chloratum* D4 – D6)
	Organ Area	
Hyperchromic anemia (lead-related); Craniotabes (*Plumbum* ointment 0.4%); Paget's disease, Sudeck's atrophy (*Plumbum silicicum* D20); Scheuermann's disease, Osgood-Schlatter disease, Perthes disease (*Cerussit* D20, *Plumbum* ointment 0.4%); Bone metastases (*Pyromorphit* D8)	Spleen; skeleton; bone marrow and hematopoiesis	Leukemia (Galenit D6, Plumbum D10); Deficient ossification, osteoporosis, osteo-malacia (Galenit D6); Osteogenesis imperfecta (*Plumbum silicicum D10, Cerussit* D8)

Tin Remedies

Area of Efficacy and Therapeutic Applications

Excessive or one-sided tin processes and corresponding remedies	Balanced tin processes and functional areas	Weak, deficient tin processes and corresponding remedies
	Soul Area	
Fear of life, inhibition of will	Balanced, measured soul life; inner equilibrium; thinks and feels things through; circumspect; actions guided by wisdom	Intoxication with life, recklessness
Hypochondria (*Taraxacum Stanno cultum* 1%);		Arrogant, domineering, imposture, pomposity, swaggering, sudden temper, manic agitation (*Stannum* D3 – D6, *Arandisit* D6);
Depression (*Arandisit* D15);		
Hallucinations, visions (*Stannum* D15);		Hepatogenic depression (*Hepar-Stannum* D4, *Stannum* D6 – D12);
Hepatogenic schizo-phrenia (*Arandisit* D15);		
Cyclothymia (*Arandisit* D15);		Poor concentration in small-headed children (*Stannum* D8)
Mental weakness in dreamy large-headed children (*Stannum* D15 – D20)		

Process and Organ Areas I.

Imbalanced transformation of peripheral formative forces with excessive tonus and drying tendency, exaggerated contour formation	Cosmic peripheral formative forces transform into metabolic forces, allowing fluidity of motion; proper relationship of plasticity and tonus, form and life; thirst regulation	Dysplasia, congestion due to inadequate tonus, deficient transformation, tendency to fluidification
Scarlet fever (*Kassiterit, extern.* liquid 0.1%);		Obesity (*Stannum* D10 – 5%);
Glaucoma (*Stannum* D20, *Stannum* D8/ *Succinum* D6aa eyedrops);		Arthritis (*Stannum* D3);
Neurodermatitis, lichen ruber planus, fissures and tears (*Stannum* D20, D30, *Taraxacum Stanno cultum* 1%);		Osteoarthritis (*Stannum* 5%);
		Flail joints (*Stannum* D6);
Cirrhosis of the liver (*Taraxacum Stanno cultum* 1%, *Stannum* D20);		Connective tissue weakness, uterine prolapse, effusions, hydrocele, edema (*Stannum* D8);
Lower back pain (*Stannum* D20);		Ovarian cysts (*Mixtura Stanni comp.*);
Multiple sclerosis (*Stannum* 5% ointment)		Megacolon (*Stannum* D6);
		Serositis, pleuritis, pericarditis (*Stannum* D10);
		Bronchitis, emphysema (*Stannum* D8);
		Hip dysplasia (*Stannum* D10)

Process and Organ Areas II.

Excessively active metabolic chemistry, conditions of tension	Metabolic chemistry, balance between solid and fluid, guidance of anabolic liver metabolism, regulation of water, regulation of swelling and shrinking	Deficient metabolic chemistry
Epilepsy (*Stannum* D20, *Arandisit D15, Stannum 0.4% ointment, Taraxacum Stanno cultum 1%*); Allergy (*Stannum* D14, D20)		Adynamia, myasthenia, psychic and physical weakness, progressive muscular atrophy (*Stannum* D3 – D6)

Organ Area

| Hydrocephalus (*Stannum* D20);

Cerebral edema (*Stannum* D20 – D30);

Migraine, weather sensitivity (*Stannum* D20 – D30);

Neuralgias, trigeminal neuralgia, neuritis (*Stannum* D20 – D30);

Cirrhosis of the liver (*Taraxacum Stanno cultum* 1%, *Stannum* D20) | Liver, serous membranes; central nervous system; musculature | Migraine, flu headache (*Stannum* D3)

Hepatopathy, hepatogenic eczema, ascites (*Stannum* D8);

Leukemia (*Galenit* D6, *Plumbum* D10);

Hepatitis (*Stannum* D6 – D8) |

Iron Remedies

Area of Efficacy and Therapeutic Applications

Excessive or one-sided iron processes and corresponding remedies	Balanced iron processes and functional areas	Weak, deficient iron processes and corresponding remedies
	Soul Area	
Overconfidence, hot-headed daredevil	Full-blooded fire type, practical, realistic mind;	No self-confidence, exhausted, pallid chlorotic type, defeated, fearful weakling
Megalomania, delusions of grandeur (*Cinis Urticae Ferro cultae* D3);	Independent and goal-oriented in actions, able to assert and control self, gifted speaker	
Hysteria, violent temper, raving madness, aggression (*Katoptrit* D20);		Nervous depressive exhaustion (*Ferrum sidereum* D6);
Chronic stress and time-pressure (*Katoptrit* D20)		Anxiety, fearful depression (*Skorodit* D6);
		Lack of will, low drive, obsessive-compulsive (*Ferrum arsenicosum* D6)

Process and Organ Areas I.

Exaggerated dynamic of inner movement directed into space	Putting one's soul dynamic into goal-oriented action toward self-assertion in space; Speaking; Circulation; Movement	Inadequate dynamic of inner movement toward self-assertion in space
Scarlet fever (*Kassiterit,* extern. liquid 0.1%); Glaucoma (*Stannum* D20, *Stannum* D8/ *Succinum* D6aa eyedrops); Neurodermatitis, lichen ruber planus, fissures and tears (*Stannum* D20, D30, *Taraxacum Stanno cultum* 1%); Cirrhosis of the liver (*Taraxacum Stanno cultum* 1%, *Stannum* D20); Lower back pain (*Stannum* D20); Multiple sclerosis (*Stannum* 5% ointment)		Circulatory lability with blood congestion in head, vascular erethism (*Ferrum* D6); Dizzy spells (*Ferrum hydroxydatum 8*); Low blood pressure (Sol. *Ferri comp.* D3, D6); Stuttering (*Pyrit* D3)

Process and Organ Areas II.

Deficient assimilation, excessive forming	Transforming, creating new order and form out of congestion	Assimilation and congestion without sufficient forming
Pruritus, hives (*Ferrum* D20);		Exaggerated protein processes, bronchitis, larygitis (*Pyrit* D3, *Ferrum phosphoricum* D6 – D8);
Allergy (*Ferrum sidereum* D20);		Colitis gravis (*Katoptrit* D6);
Asthma with mucous obstruction (*Nontronit* D15);		Flu (*Ferrum phosphoricum* D6);
Encephalitis, meningitis (*Ferrum sidereum* D20);		Migraine (*Biodoron*);
Pemphigus (*Urtica dioica Ferro culta* 1%)		Pulmonary tuberculosis, exud. (*Ferrum phosphoricum* D6);
		Varices, hemorrhoids (*Haematit* D6, *Skorodit* D10);
		Articular rheumatism (*Haematit* D6)
	Organ Area	
	Gallbladder, larynx; Blood circulation; Warmth organization; Hematopoiesis	Biliary disorders, acholia, cholecystitis (*Chelidonium Ferro cultum* 1%);
		Hepatitis (*Ferrum* D6);
		Iron deficiency anemia (*Haematit* D6);
		Anemia in pregnancy (*Ferrum pomatum* D1, *Ferrum ustum comp.*)

Gold Remedies

Area of Efficacy and Therapeutic Applications

Excessive or one-sided gold processes and corresponding remedies	Balanced gold processes and functional areas	Weak, deficient gold processes and corresponding remedies
	Soul Area	
Darkening of soul through self-centered entrenchment in the spatial confines of the material world.	Vital, full-blooded, socially engaged pyknic; choleric temperament; positivity, openness, idealism, trust in life; courageous, sincere, enthusiastic	Loosening of soul due to excessive extroversion
Obsessive-compulsive disorder, self-reproach, anxiety, depression (*Aurum* D15 – D30, *Mercurius auratus* D15);		Mania, agitation, raving (*Aurum* D6 – D10);
Sense of confinement, claustrophobia (*Hypericum Auro cultum* 0.1%);		Expansive urge, euphoria (*Aurum* D4 – D6);
Danger of suicide (*Aurum* D20 – D30);		Schizophrenia (*Aurum D6/Stibium* D6);
Autism (*Myrrha comp.*)		Violent temper (*Aurum* D4 – D6);
		Anxiety, lack of trust in life (*Aurum* D12 – D15)

Process and Organ Areas I.

Rigidity of inner center, constriction, solidification	Expansion – contraction, diastole – systole; Creating a functional equilibrium and inner center	Loss of inner center Dizziness, fainting, depressed level of consciousness
Stenocardia, angina pectoris (*Aurum* D30); Heart attack, hypertension with plethora (*Aurum* D30); Acute psychogenic erythma (*Primula Auro culta* 0.1%); Renal congestion, chronic nephritis (*Aurum* D15); Nephrosclerosis (*Aurum* D20 – D30)		Low blood pressure and venous congestion (*Aurum* D6 – D10); Vegetative circulatory disorders (*Aurum* D10); Palpitations, cardiac neurosis, extrasystole, tachycardia, cardiac arrhythmia (*Aurum* D10, *Stibium* D8); Graves' disease (*Aurum* D10); Weather sensitivity (*Aurum* D10/*Stibium* D8 /*Hyoscyamus* D5)

Process and Organ Areas II.

Uncontrolled destruction, excessive breakdown, solidification, hardening	Materialization and spiritualization, solidifying and dissolving; anabolism and catabolism in equilibrium	Bone metastases (*Aurum D20 – D30*) Uncontrolled hypertrophy, excessive releasing and dissolving tendency
Autoaggressive diseases, lupus vulgaris (*Aurum* D15, *Aurum* D5 ointment); Sclerosis (*Aurum* D20/ *Betula Cortex* D2); Multiple sclerosis (*Aurum* D30); Dry, itchy exzema, flaky keratosis, erythema nodosum, neurodermatitis (*Aurum* D15 – D30); Cysts and fibromas of the thyroid, breast and genitals (*Aurum* D20 – D30); Sun allergy (*Aurum* D30)		Chronic inflammation of the mucous membranes, glands, and genitals (*Aurum* D6 – D10); Carditis, arteritis, aortitis (*Aurum* D15); Rosacea (*Aurum* D5 ointment); Increased cutaneous blood, erythema (*Aurum* D4 – D10); Infectious hepatitis and cirrhosis of the liver (*Aurum* D6)
	Organ Area	
Cardiac myodegeneration (*Aurum* D20 – D30); Benign genital tumors (fibroma of uterus, myoma, prostate hypertrophy) (*Aurum* D20 – D30)	Heart, circulation, genitals	Imminent abortion (*Aurum* D6); Genital hypoplasia, chronic inflammation of the genitals (*Aurum* D6, D8)

Copper Remedies

Area of Efficacy and Therapeutic Applications

Excessive or one-sided copper processes and corresponding remedies	Balanced copper processes and functional areas	Weak, deficient copper processes and corresponding remedies
	Soul Area	
Addiction to the body, soul fever	Loving, devoted, careful, thrifty, gracious, tactful;	Fear of the body, coldness of soul
Slave to emotional desire-nature, narcissism, autism, schizophrenia, schizophrenic hallucinations (*Dioptas* D20);	Caring for and tending to others, altruistic, empathetic, full of longing;	Apathy, dullness, infantilism, phobias (*Cuprum* D6);
	Sanguinic temperament;	Stuttering (*Cuprum aceticum* D3 – D6);
Kleptomania (*Cuprum* D30);	Analogical image-based thinking;	Depression (*Cuprum* D6)
Hysteria (*Cuprum* ointment 0.4%);	Sense of beauty	
Agitation accompanying hypertension (*Chamomilla Cupro culta* 1%)		

Process and Organ Areas I.

Excessive sheath and boundary formation, impairment of inner space	Creating a receptive space and sheath for that which is higher, healing, beautiful, perfect	Inadequate sheath and boundary formation, insufficient creation of inner space, congestion
Cramping, dystonia, pylorospasm (*Chamomilla Cupro culta* 1%, *Cuprum* ointment 0.4%);		Loosening, atonia, Graves' disease (*Cuprit* D3, *Chalkosin* D3);
Calf cramps (*Cuprum* D30);		Tachykardia (*Cuprit* D6);
Epilepsy (*Cuprum* D20/ *Chamomilla* D30);		Vegetative dystonia (*Malachit* D6);
Nephrogenic hypertension (*Olivenit* D30);		Ptosis, esophageal diverticula (*Cuprum sulfuricum* D6);
Constipation (*Cuprum* ointment 0.4%);		Varices, hemorrhoids, varicosis, (*Cuprum* D6/ *Urtica dioica* D3aa);
Bronchial asthma, spastic bronchitis (*Tabacum Cupro cultum* 0.1%)		Grimacing, head nodding, muscle twitches, ticks (*Cuprum aceticum* D3);
		Spasmophilia (*Cuprum aceticum* D3 – D6)

Process and Organ Areas II.

Excessive excretion	Nutrition, assimilation, secretion and excretion; **Growth**	Inadequate excretion
Cachexia (*Cuprum* D15); Vitiligo (*Cuprum* 0.4% ointment); Alopecia, digestion and absorption disorders (*Melissa Cupro culta* 1%); Exhaustion with apathy, hypotension, chills (*Melissa Cupro culta* 1%)		Adiposity, gout, exzema (*Cuprum* D8); Allergy, hives (*Chalkopyrit* D6)
	Organ Area	
Nephritis, atrophic kidney (*Cuprum* 0.4% ointment)	Kidney, thyroid	Atrophic kidney (*Olivenit* D6 – D8); Nephrosis (*Olivenit* D6); Uremia (*Olivenit* D10); Graves' disease (*Cuprit* D3, *Chalkosin* D3)

Mercury Remedies

Area of Efficacy and Therapeutic Applications

Excessive or one-sided mercury processes and corresponding remedies	Balanced mercury processes and functional areas	Weak, deficient mercury processes and corresponding remedies
	Soul Area	
Restlessness, agitation;	Mobile, sanguinic, slender Mercury-type;	Sluggish, phlegmatic, lymphatic, adenoid patient
Fidgety, rushed, distracted neurasthenic	Intelligent, logical thinking;	
	Extroverted personality;	"Clinginess," obsessive-compulsive neurosis, obsessive ideas, compulsive actions, pathological egocentricity
Hysteria, mania (*Bryophyllum Mercurio cultum* 1%);	Acts as a mediator;	
	Capacity for meeting, humor;	
Delusions, depression with compulsion neurosis (*Mercurius auratus* D15);	Capacity for change;	Dullness, clumsiness (*Mercurius vivus nat.* D6)
	Stability;	
Logorrhea, erethism mercurialis (*Bryophyllum Mercurio cultum* 1%)	Self-contained	

Process and Organ Areas I.

Circulation of fluids too lively, foreign matter is not warded off, exchange or mediation does not take place	Circulation of fluids (lymph);	Fluid circulation too sluggish, deception instead of exchange, failure to recognize or eliminate what is foreign
Allergies (*Nasturtium Mercurio cultu* 0.1%);	**Transformation and mediation through plastic formation of meeting streams;**	Edema, congestion, lymphangitis (*Mercurialis bijodatum* D4, *Mercurius dulcis* D4);
Hodgkin's lymphoma (*Mercurius vivus nat.* D15 – D30);	**Recognition of self and other;**	Lymphedema (*Mercurius vivus nat.* D8, *Mercurius dulcis* D4);
Cardiac insufficiency, cardiac asthma (*Mercurius vivus nat.* D15 – D30);	**Exchange**	Tachykardia, heat exhaustion (*Mercurius vivus nat.* D10);
Congestive headaches (*Mercurius vivus nat.* D20 – D30)		Nephrosis (*Mercurius vivus nat.* D6);
		Mumps (*Mercurius vivus nat.* D8)

Process and Organ Areas II.

Excessive binding, hypertrophy of the cells	Binding and releasing; Structuring toward the inside, secreting and releasing to the outside; Manifesting the spiritual through transformation; Exercising a threshold function	Inadequate structuring toward the inside, secreting to the outside, excessively dissolving
Fibroma, myoma, prostatic hypertrophy (*Mercurius auratus* D15/*Helleborus niger* D4); Papilloma, mastopathy, adenoma (*Mercurius vivus nat.* D15 – D30)		Hypersecretion, inflammation, mucosal inflammation of oral cavity and colon (*Mercurius sol. D6, Mercurius vivus nat. D8, Mercurius vivus comp.*); Laryngitis (*Zinnober* D6); Hepatitis (*Mercurius dulcis* D6); Colitis (*Mercurius sublimatus corrosivus* D6); Cholecystitis (*Mercurius vivus nat. D6*); Nephritis (*Mercurius corrosivus* D4 – D6)
	Soul Area	
Lymphogranulo-matosis; Hodgkin's lymphoma (*Mercurius vivus nat.* D15 – D30)	Lungs, glands, mucosae	Lymphangitis (*Mercurius bijodatus* D4); Diphtheria, swelling of lymph nodes, mumps (*Mercurius vivus nat. D8*)

Silver Remedies

Area of Efficacy and Therapeutic Applications

Excessive or one-sided silver processes and corresponding remedies	Balanced silver processes and functional areas	Weak, deficient silver processes and corresponding remedies
	Soul Area	
Living in a world of illusory images (media, glamor)	Imaginative, moral imagination; Independent thinker; Rich feeling and thought life, thoughtful, healthy sense of family, warm motherliness, creative capacities	Lacking moral imagination; intellectual, dry soul life
Visionary disposition, hallucinations, endogenous psychosis, hysteria (*Dyskrasit* D20, *Bryophyllum Argento cultum* 0.1%); Psychological loosening (*Argentum* D20 – D30); Pregnancy psychosis, climacteric psychosis (*Argentum* D20); Restless, rushed (*Bryophyllum Argento cultum* 01%)		Unimaginative; intellectually precocious (mostly in small-headed children); inner aridity, depression (*Argentit* D6, *Argentum* D6); Somnambulism, hysterogenic depressive mood, sensation of head expanding (*Argentit* D6); Rushed, always in a hurry, anxiety, compulsive ideas (*Argentum* D6)

Process and Organ Areas I.

Exaggerated silver process in the metabolic area, weak action of the nerve-sense system

Obesity
(*Argentum* D30);

Hot flashes in climacteric
(*Dyskrasit* D20);

Left side migraine with gradual onset and sudden cessation, neurasthenic migraine
(*Argentum* D20);

Epilepsy
(*Argentum* D20 – D30);

Enuresis (*Argentum* 0.4% ointment)

Creating "copies," replicating images, developing form;

Promoting regeneration and physical recovery;

Regulation and structuring of the water organism

Nerve-sense (silver) process displaced into the metabolic area, weak anabolic activity in the metabolism

Sleep disorders
(*Argentum D8/ Hyoscyamus* D3 aa);

Shock (*Argentum* D6, *Argentit* D6);

Prolapse of the gastro-intestinal tract
(*Argentum* D6);

Vegetative dystonia, general vegetative irritability; stomach neurosis (nervous dyspepsia), gastritis, stomach ulcer
(*Argentum* D6, *Argentum nitricum* D6);

Sugar intolerance
(*Argentum* D6);

Bedwetting
(*Argentum* D6)

Process and Organ Areas II.

Too strong catabolism and too strong excretion	Anabolism and excretion in balance; Secretion and differentiation; Structuring of anabolic metabolic processes	Too weak anabolism, deficient structuring and differentiation
Fever, sepsis (*Argentum* D20, *Argentum* D30/ *Echinacea* D6 aa);		Cachexia (*Argentit* D6, *Argentum nitricum* D4);
Lochial congestion (*Argentum* D20);		Sinusitis, stomatitis (*Argentus nitricum* D4, D6);
Chronic inflammations, purulence (*Argentum* D20 – D30);		Diarrhea/constipation, ulcerative colitis (*Argentum nitricum* D4, D6);
Periodontosis, alveolar pyorrhea (*Argentum nitricum* D20 – D30)		Urethritis, cystitis, pyelonephritis (*Argentum nitricum* D6);
		Acute inflammations, furuncles, paronychia, abscesses, phlegmons (*Argentum D6, Argentit* D4 – D6)

Soul Area

Neuralgia in the head region (*Argentum* D20)	Reproductive organs; central nervous system, mucosae; skin	Conception difficulties, sterility, repeated miscarriage (*Argentum* D6);
		Dysmenorrhea, uterine hypoplasia (*Argentit* D6);
		Vaginal discharge (*Argentum* D6)

PHOTO CREDITS

Figures 1 through 7 represent the planetary seals as executed by Justina Schachenmann-Teichert based on Rudolf Steiner's drawings. For further information, see Rudolf Steiner, *Kleinodienkunst als goetheanistische Formensprache* (GA K 51), Rudolf Steiner Verlag, Dornach/Schweiz, 1984. The seals are customarily placed in a different order than they appear in our study because of contrasting approaches to the planetary levels. When these differences are considered, the seals can make impressions that correspond to the material presented.

Figures 8 through 14 are taken from *Der astrologische Gedanke in der deutschen Vergangenheit* by Heinz Artur Strauss, Verlag A. Oldenburg, Munich and Berlin, 1926. They come from a medieval compendium dating to 1480 and were implemented as prints by H. L. Petersen.

BIBLIOGRAPHY

Bauer, S. W., J. Dunat, S. Golowin. *Lexikon der Symbole*. Wiesbaden: Fourier Verlag, 1980.

Beckh, Hermann. *Alchymie. Vom Geheimnis der Stoffeswelt*, 4th ed. Dornach: Rudolf Geering Verlag, 1987.

Benesch, Friedrich. *Apokalypse*. Stuttgart: Verlag Urachhaus, 1981.

Boegner, Karl. *Es war einmal—die Entstehung der Grimmschen Märchen*. Dornach, Switzerland: Verlag am Goetheanum, 1988.

Capra, Fritjof. *The Tao of Physics*. Boston: Shambhala, 1999.

Cooper, J. C. *An Illustrated Encyclopaedia of Traditional Symbols*. Thames and Hudson, 1987.

Grimm, Hermann. *Household Stories by the Brothers Grimm*. New York: Dover, 1963.

Holm-Hadulla, Michael. *Psychologische Aspekte der Krebskerkrankung*. Göttingen: Verlag für medizinische Psychologie, 1982.

Jung, C. G. *Man and His Symbols*. New York: Dell, 1964.

Köhler, Gerhard. *Handbook of Homeopathy*. Rochester VT: Healing Arts Press, 1989.

Lievegoed, Bernard. *Man on the Threshold*. Stroud, UK: Hawthorn Press, 1996.

Lorenzen, Iwer Thor. *Metamorphosen*. Hamburg: Verlag für zeitgemäßen Goetheanismus, 1958.

Meyer, Rudolf. *The Wisdom of Fairy Tales*. Edinburgh: Floris Books, 1995.

Roger, Bernard. *A la découverte de l'alchimie*. Edition Dangles, St-Jean-de-Braye, France, 1988.

Rölleke, Heinz. *Kinder- und Hausmärchen, gesammelt durch die Brüder Grimm*. Göttingen: Verlag Vandenhoeck and Ruprecht, 1986.

Schult, Arthur. *Maria Sophia. Das ewig Weibliche in Gott, Mensch und Kosmos*. Bietigheim/Württemberg: Turm Verlag, 1986.

Selawry Alla. *Metallfunktionstypen in Psychologie und Medizin*. Heidelberg: Haug Verlag, 1985.

Steiner, Rudolf. *At Home in the Universe: Exploring Our Suprasensory Nature*. Hudson, NY: Anthroposophic Press, 2000.

———. *Background to the Gospel of St. Mark*. London: Rudolf Steiner Press, 1968.

———. *The Christian Mystery*. Hudson, NY: Anthroposophic Press, 1998.

———. *Color.* London: Rudolf Steiner Press, 1992.

———. *Education for Special Needs: The Curative Education Course.* London: Rudolf Steiner Press, 1999.

———. *Ergebnisse der Geistesforschung.* Basel: Rudolf Steiner Verlag, 1989.

———. *Eurythmy as Visible Speech.* London: Rudolf Steiner Press, 1984.

———. *Foundations of Esotericism.* London: Rudolf Steiner Press, 1983.

———. *From Comets to Cocaine...: Answers to Questions.* London: Rudolf Steiner Press, 2001.

———. *From Elephants to Einstein...: Answers to Questions.* London: Rudolf Steiner Press, 1999.

———. *Das Geheimnis des Todes. Wesen und Bedeutung Mitteleuropas und die europäischen Volksgeister.* Basel: Rudolf Steiner Verlag, 2005.

———. *Harmony of the Creative Word: The Human Being and the Elemental, Animal, Plant, and Mineral Kingdoms.* London: Rudolf Steiner Press, 2001.

———. *The Healing Process: Spirit, Nature and Our Bodies.* Great Barrington, MA: SteinerBooks, 2010.

———. *The Human Soul in Relation to World Evolution.* Spring Valley, NY: Anthroposophic Press, 1984.

———. *The Influence of Spiritual Beings on Man.* Spring Valley, NY: Anthroposophic Press, 1961.

———. *Initiationswissenschaft und Sternenerkenntnis.* Basel: Rudolf Steiner Verlag, 1964.

———. *Introducing Anthroposophical Medicine.* Great Barrington, MA: SteinerBooks, 1999.

———. *Macrocosm and Microcosm.* London: Rudolf Steiner Press, 1986.

———. *Der Mensch in Zusammenhang mit dem Kosmos.* Basel: Rudolf Steiner Verlag, 1981.

———. *Die Mission der neuen Geistesoffenbarung. Das Christus-Ereignis als Mittelpunktsgeschehen der Erdenevolution.* Basel: Rudolf Steiner Verlag, 1975.

———. *Mystery Knowledge and Mystery Centres.* London: Rudolf Steiner Press, 2013.

———. *Mystery of the Universe: The Human Being, Model of Creation.* London: Rudolf Steiner Press, 2001.

———. *An Occult Physiology.* London: Rudolf Steiner Press, 2005.

———. *Physiologisch-Therapeutisches auf Grundlage der Geisteswissenschaft: Zur Therapie und Hygiene* (Physiological Therapeutics). Basel: Rudolf Steiner Verlag, 2011.

———. *An Outline of Esoteric Science.* Hudson, NY: Anthroposophic Press, 1997.

———. *The Riddle of Man.* Spring Valley, NY: Mercury Press, 1990.

———. *Spiritual Beings in the Heavenly Bodies and in the Kingdoms of Nature.* Great Barrington, MA: SteinerBooks, 2012.

———. *True and False Paths in Spiritual Investigation.* London: Rudolf Steiner Press, 1985.

———. *Der Zusammenhang des Menschen mit der elementarischen Welt. Kalewala—Olaf Åsteson—Das russische Volkstum—Die Welt als Ergebnis von Gleichgewichtswirkungen.* Basel: Rudolf Steiner Verlag, 1993.

Tylor Kent, J. T. *Arzneimittelbilder—Vorlesungen zur homöopathischen Materia Medica.* Ulm, 1958.